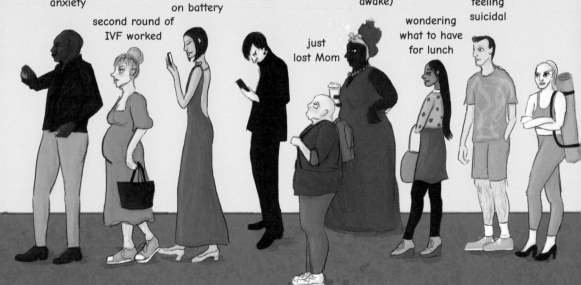

WHY AREN'T WE TALKING ABOUT THIS?!

First published in the US in 2024 by Interlink Books
An imprint of Interlink Publishing Group, Inc.
46 Crosby Street, Northampton, Massachusetts 01060
www.interlinkbooks.com

"Sex is So Much More Than PIV" (page 31–2) was originally commissioned by The
Vaginismus Network, "A Celebration of the Underrated Kiss" was originally commissioned
by The Sex School Hub, "Postpartum Bodies" (page 187–8) was originally commissioned
by Elvie, and "UTIs" (page 70) was originally commissioned by Velive.

Page design by maru studio
Cover design by Mylène Mozas
Editor: Nina Shield

Library of Congress Cataloging-in-Publication Data available
ISBN-13: 978-1-62371-696-7 (hardback)

Printed and bound in Korea
10 9 8 7 6 5 4 3 2 1

This book does not replace medical attention from qualified practitioners. Please consult
your primary care physician or psychologist before starting any serious course of treatment.

Interlink Publishing Group is committed to a sustainable future for our business, our readers
and our planet.
This book is made from Forest Stewardship Council® certified paper.

WHY AREN'T WE TALKING ABOUT THIS?!

Hazel Mead

An Inclusive Guide to Life, Love, Sex, and Identity in 100+ Questions

Interlink Books
An imprint of Interlink Publishing Group, Inc.

Contents

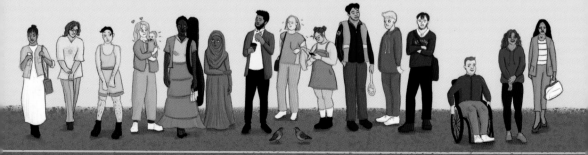

HEALTH + WELLBEING 95

THE SELF + SOCIETY 163

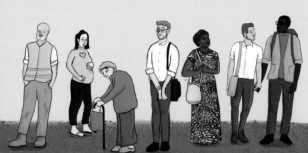

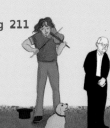

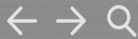

Banana + Condom + Shame = Sex Ed

What was the most important thing you learned in school? Be honest: how much of your formative schooling do you *truly* remember? When was the last time you used the Pythagorean theorem, $E=mc^2$, or iambic pentameter at work, at home or . . . in the bedroom? (To any mathematicians, physicists, or poets reading this: I see you. And I can absolutely see how poetry may help with the "bedroom" bit!)

In fairness, even though biology was not my cup of tea, for others photosynthesis ignited their passion. And while they might have despised drawing, I loved art so much that it became my entire career. But there was one small lesson that was missed in my own (and many loved ones') core education, and that's, well, everything to do with life.

While I left school feeling extremely well versed in the marital relations of King Henry VIII, I felt unprepared to deploy the requisite skills to navigate my relationships, my health, or any wider understanding of society. Sex was reduced to a matter-of-fact overview of the biology of what's happening inside various cells, and how to put a condom on a banana, peppered with a dollop of shame and judgment, warning against it. There was nothing about pleasure or the emotional side of sex. Relationships, mental health, sexuality, coping with grief, the effects of technology on us, identity—very large factors in everyone's life—were barely explored, or at best were crammed into a lesson taught by your homeroom teacher, who clearly felt uncomfortable advising on something beyond their usual realm. Thankfully, curriculums are slowly changing and these topics are being given some acknowledgment. Perhaps it was easier to suppress these complex topics—but "easier" for whom?

Inspired by the many things I wish I had been taught in school, I want to collate some of the key life lessons that, although I have found to be the most important, have not been given the same attention as academic lessons and are often omitted

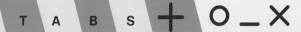

T A B S

from, or glossed over in, core educational establishments across the world. I'm an illustrator and a visual storyteller, focusing my work on the human experience, which often crosses into some so-called taboo topics. What I've found, through opening up to friends and sharing my personal illustrations with the world, is that conversations about difficult topics can make you feel far less alone. Perhaps what you perceive to be your oddities are simply part of being human and are much more common than you think—we just don't talk about them.

However, with the internet at our fingertips, while we may still struggle to turn to close ones for answers, we can turn to search engines, forums, and strangers instead. Google's top search trends provide fascinating reading and give an insight into what is capturing the minds of the majority (among those who have internet access). Many of the top searched-for questions that I came

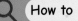

How to

TOP HITS
- How to be happy
- How to kiss
- How to love yourself
- How to have sex
- How to last longer in bed
- How to be single
- How to get over a breakup
- How to make pancakes
- How to cut a mango
- Maintaining mental health
- Body positivity
- Doomscrolling
- Soulmates
- Can you get pregnant on your period?
- Does he like me?
- Why is my poop green?
- When does the time change?
- What is a virtual private network/VPN?
- What is the meaning of life?

across while writing this book inevitably revolved around the pandemic, although search trends from recent years perhaps reveal something more eternal.

While many searches revolve around briefly trending topics, or how to prepare certain food, many others speak to more global concerns.

"Maintaining mental health" is at an all-time high, as are **"affirmations"**—positive words or phrases that we repeat to ourselves to enhance our self-belief. If the effects of a whole world experiencing a pandemic and having to isolate, not seeing loved ones or being allowed outside, and witnessing large-scale death have shown us anything, it's how important mental health—as well as physical health—is. Finally we're taking our mental health a bit more seriously, although there's still a long way to go.

The themes of **"lasting longer in bed"** and **"how to make love"** reflect the insecurities shining through in so many people, and perhaps a yearning to connect and be deemed a "good" lover, as a result of insufficient sex education.

Newer searches, such as **"doomscrolling"** and **"What is a virtual private network?"**, speak to the digital age that we find ourselves in. The fast growth of this technological revolution brings both new opportunities and new dangers to navigate, in terms of digital security and guarding mental health.

Perhaps the most existential and eternal search-question is **"What is the meaning of life?"** It calls into question our identity, ego, and purpose, and our attempts to understand how to do something meaningful with our brief, but cherished, time here.

This book weaves together life lessons I wish I'd learned earlier with answers to the essential questions that we have collectively most asked Google in recent years.

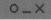

ABOUT THIS BOÖK

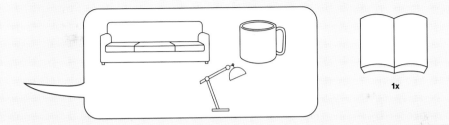

1x

This book is a collection of illustrations that I hope will shine a light on topics that are generally not discussed, as well as diagrams that will demystify how things work. I've included interviews with experts, to help make sense of some complex themes, and have included frameworks that I find helpful in day-to-day life, as well as research and advice from some incredible organizations.

It's important to note that this book is an introduction to many ideas, but by the end I hope you will have food for thought on how to navigate this complicated, messy human life, as well as a few practical tips to help you through. Read the whole thing from cover to cover, pop in and out, start with any section; look at all the illustrations first, if that's your thing; or read the bits that you need, as and when you experience them. Some parts may become relevant to you in the future; other parts may no longer be applicable to you.

I have separated the ideas into three sections—relationships + sex, health + wellbeing, the self + society—all of which explore different ideas and theories and offer practical tips. I'd love this book to be a conversation starter and to bring some taboo topics into the mainstream. Rather than being intended as an all-inclusive resource (as I realize that I can't speak for the nearly eight billion of us on this planet), I hope this book can serve as a jumping-off point into some of these crucial topics. I want this to be the resource that every person who is sixteen or older can turn to while they're figuring out these essential and yet marginalized subjects, so that they feel less alone on their quest.

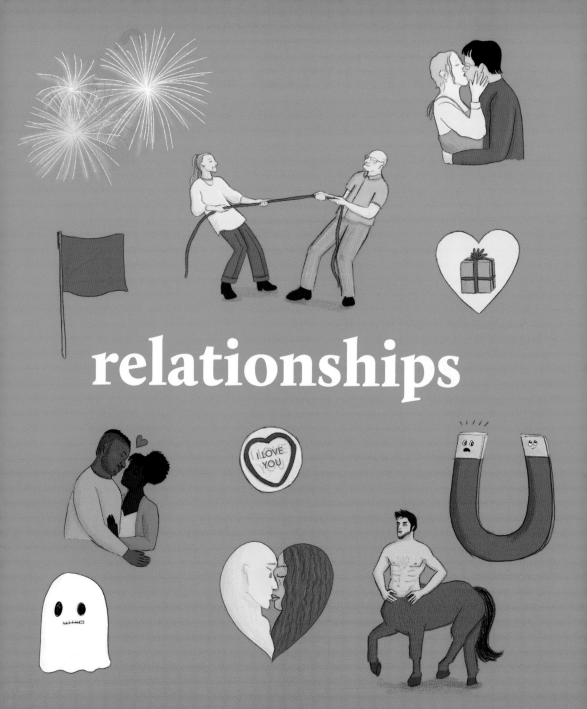

relationships

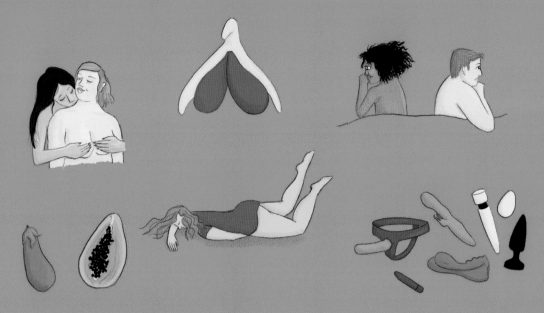

+ sex

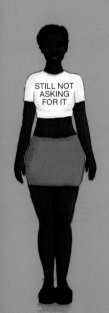

STILL NOT ASKING FOR IT

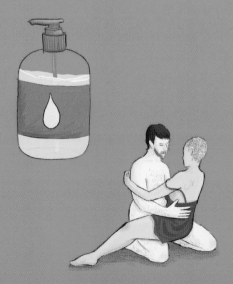

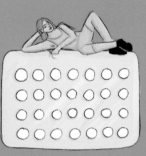

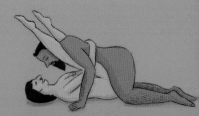

Throughout history, humans have survived by forming relationships (familial, platonic, romantic, and sexual), so no wonder we seek them out, agonize over them, write songs and lamentations about them—that's been a constant for thousands of years.

Relationships are notoriously tricky things to manage, with two—and sometimes more—sets of egos, opinions, and minds trying to come together to create something that works for everyone. And we never have any formal training, probably because we're fickle, unpredictable, emotional, and messy beings, so there isn't a one-size-fits-all method. We learn from parents, close ones, and different influences around us how to behave in relationships. Our experiences of how we've been treated can impact the way we treat others, and whether we recreate or reject what we have experienced ourselves.

Sex is another messy topic. For many of us, our sex life is a place where we can explore our most vulnerable side with someone else, and that's part of what makes it so taboo (not to mention the many moralistic connotations it's often wrapped up in). Due to this sensitive nature, we rarely get education on the emotional intricacies of sex.

Let's explore the parts of sex ed that may have been left out and along the way address those common sex and relationships myths that may have made you feel bad about your desires, boundaries, or experiences.

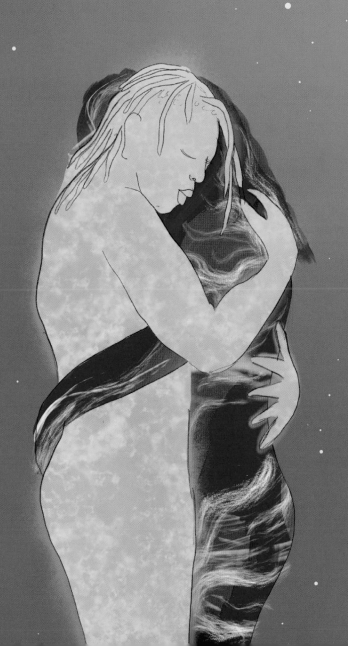

DATING GAMES

PLAYING HARD TO GET

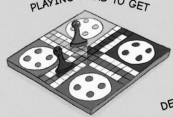

RULES: 4 DATES BEFORE GETTING A HOTEL

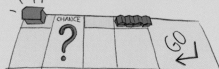

NO SEX ON THE FIRST DATE

DECIPHERING CRYPTIC TEXT MESSSAGES

KEEPING YOUR CARDS CLOSE TO YOUR CHEST

ACROSS

1. Thinking of getting this top, what do you think?

ACROSS

2. Can't sleep, do you want to come over and have pizza? 02:00

DOWN

1. We should see other people

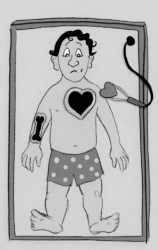

STEALING HEARTS

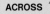

	T	E	L	L		M	E		H	O	W
	G	O	O	D		I		L	O	O	K
						M					
	P	R	O	B	A	B	L	E			
	H	O	O	K	U	P					
						R					
						E					
						D					

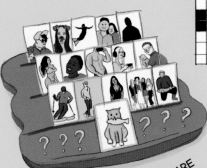

GUESS WHO THEY ARE
UNDER THE DATING PROFILE

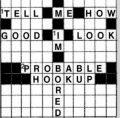

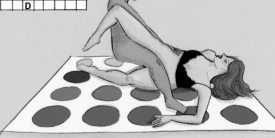

BRINGING OUT YOUR BEST MOVES

WHY IS DATING SO DIFFICULT?

If dating feels hard to you, you're not alone. While there's excitement and possibility, it may also feel demoralizing at times. With the widespread use of dating apps, we have access to so many more people in the world. Additionally, travel is much more common than it used to be. Whereas previous generations were more likely to stay and marry someone from their hometown, we increasingly have more options, and our dating pool is much bigger.

With this vast amount of choice comes the thinking, "What if there is someone better out there for me?"—and you're not satisfied with "great" because you're looking for "impeccable." Our expectations are higher, and that's not a bad thing—for example, no one should accept someone who treats them poorly.

However, when it comes to having a rigid list of physical qualities that you expect in another person, everyone suffers the consequences. Let's face it, people often have superficial criteria on dating apps—for instance, "Must be blonde, petite, skinny, big boobs" or "Don't message me if you're under six feet tall."

Dating apps also offer convenience. You can talk to people from the comfort of your own home, in your pajamas, and be, well, lazy about it. If someone starts boring you, there are eight other matches you can talk to—perhaps you're already talking to six of them. People start becoming commodities—and you know that's how people are treating you, too.

Dating games and unwritten dating rules often come into play— "treat 'em mean, keep 'em keen," "wait a few hours before texting back," etc.—to maintain some sort of power balance. While it can be a lot of fun, it can often be a minefield looking for your partner(s), and understandably many people flip-flop from installing dating apps to deleting again, from actively searching to actively not searching.

WHY ARE RELATIONSHIPS SO DIFFICULT?: LOSS OF FREEDOM VS CRAVING SECURITY

A common concern in romantic relationships (and elsewhere in life, to be honest) is feeling a loss of freedom and identity, especially once the novelty of a relationship wears off and the realities set in. Some people crave more security, while others crave more freedom and escape. Once we reconcile ourselves to the fact that our partner may need a little more of one or the other, then we can accommodate it and work to find a better balance. A feeling of loss of freedom can occur when entering new relationships, becoming a parent, or taking on more responsibilities. If you feel like you no longer have time for your hobbies and interests, discuss this with your partner and actively agree on a little alone-time each week or month—and find out what your partner would like, too. While this is much easier said than done amid all the responsibilities, work, family, and chores, it can help some people to retain a sense of personal identity.

IDEA

RELATIONSHIP CHECK-IN!

Have a date to discuss what's working, what might not be, and to see how the other person *really* feels. Just make sure it sounds like a fun time together, so that you don't freak out your beloved.

THE SLOG OF MONOGAMY

While as animals we pair-bond, we're not hardwired to be monogamous, so one person for life is a tough ask. Monogamy was invented with the rise of agriculture (see page 30), to simplify land and money inheritance decisions. While marriage was historically a financial arrangement, nowadays we have developed romantic notions of "the one"—one person who loves us completely, meets our sexual desires, with whom we can share our deepest secrets, who understands us, who will fulfill and complete us, and be our emotional crutch, our roommate, and possibly a co-parent. It's a lot to ask of one person. Those classic tales of "happily ever after" often focus on the lead-up to being in a relationship, and omit the challenges and struggles of the day-to-day, long-term relationship.

While monogamy is hard, it doesn't mean ethical non-monogamy—being romantically/sexually involved with more than one person with consent from all parties involved—is easy.

It is not about cheating, as everyone involved should be fully aware and agree to what is happening; rather, it is a relationship structure that acknowledges that as creatures we might struggle with monogamy, and allows for exploration of more than one partner. It doesn't mean cheating and jealousy don't happen, and it requires just as much care as a monogamous relationship, with more sets of feelings (and schedules) to manage.

Whatever your relationship structure, by nature relationships require work and compromise.

TI AMO

KOCHAM CIĘ

E AROHA ANA AHAU KI A KOE

あなたが好きです

WHAT IS MY LOVE LANGUAGE?

JE T'AIME

IK HOU VAN JE

AMO-TE

SZERETLEK

One place to start the work is through the rather sweet framework of love languages. The concept was first developed in 1992 by the Christian author and counselor Gary Chapman. They refer to the ways in which we prefer to give and receive love— and the concept taps into our desire to understand ourselves and our relationships. We're not always great at communicating and can misinterpret what the other person likes, by basing our ideas on our own preferences or assumptions rather than asking them. Love languages can provide a helpful guide to begin thinking about how we like to be loved, how we can express that to a partner, and how we can love our partners in a way that makes them feel loved, too.

JAG ÄLSKAR DIG

MI YIDIMA

EU TE AMO

ANH YEU EM

أنا أحبك

ICH LIEBE DICH

我愛你

ASAVAKKIT

사랑해요

I LOVE YOU

JEG ELSKER DEG

NA KIRINLA GAGUIDOU

MAIN TUMSE PYAR KARTA HUN

TIAKO IANAO

THE FIVE TYPES
OF LOVE LANGUAGE

WORDS OF AFFIRMATION

Praise, compliments, encouragement, and appreciation. For example, a grateful thank you, a compliment on appearance, or encouragement to do something.

GIFTS

A physical symbol of love—something thoughtful, a token of appreciation, proof that someone was thinking about you.

QUALITY TIME

Getting undivided attention through good conversation and time really spent together. For instance, spending time phone-free, in an activity to bond over, together.

ACTS OF SERVICE

Doing practical things that you know will be helpful or nice. For example, fixing something around the house, helping with a chore when the other person is tired, restocking the toilet paper, cooking a meal, or making a hot drink.

PHYSICAL TOUCH

Physical contact that brings you closer together. For instance, cuddles, holding hands, sex, or stroking.

To figure out which types of love language you and your partner like best, ask each other:

- What have previous relationships missed?
- What do you crave more of in this relationship?
- What love language resonates the most with you?

I like to think of love languages as a springboard for how I like to receive love.

I would also add that one of my personal love languages is silliness and laughter, so you can venture out of the framework.

It can also be applied to close friends, family, and even yourself.

LOVE THYSELF!

GIFTS

A book that you've been eyeing · Sweet treats · A new item of clothing · A trip away

QUALITY TIME

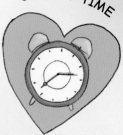

Hobbies · Reading · Walks · Setting boundaries · Solo dates

WORDS OF AFFIRMATION

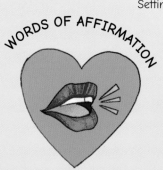

Journaling · Positive self-talk · Gratitude lists · Motivational quotes stuck on the wall

ACTS OF SERVICE

Planning · Organizing/decluttering · Therapy · Doing something that your future self would be grateful for

PHYSICAL TOUCH

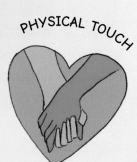

Baths · Massages/pampering · Moving your body/yoga/gym

WHAT IS AN ATTACHMENT STYLE?

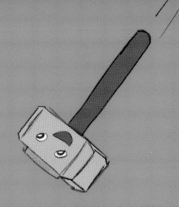

In relationships, do you find you're drawn to the same type of people? Or perhaps you've been told by partners that you're too "clingy" or too "cold"? Attachment theory offers some answers as to why we act in certain ways in relationships. Attachment theory stems from clinical psychologist John Bowlby's idea that the relationships formed in the first few years of life, between the primary caregiver and the child, set the precedent for behavior in relationships later on.

The psychologist Mary Ainsworth expanded on Bowlby's theory with her own experiments and discovered three styles of attachment: **secure, anxious,** and **avoidant.** Later, the psychologist Mary Main discovered one more: **disorganized.** Perhaps you're a mix of some of these styles, and it can be useful to think of this topic as a spectrum instead of as boxes, as they're not fixed and it's possible to exhibit behaviors of each. Being aware of how these styles are formed, and how they present themselves, can help you understand yourself in your relationships.

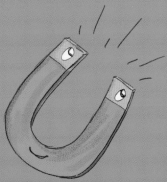

ANXIOUS

This is believed to be formed by getting inconsistent care as an infant—perhaps one minute you're shown care, then the next being ignored for some reason, and will crave the care previously exhibited.

- You may worry that you're not loved.
- You may fear the end of a relationship.
- You may feel uncomfortable being single.
- You may need constant reassurance in relationships.
- You may have a negative view of yourself.
- You may be a great caregiver to loved ones.
- People may have called you "clingy" or "needy" on occasion.

DISORGANIZED

This is believed to be formed by experiencing either frightening behavior or role confusion (where you may have had to take on the role of the parent) as an infant and young child.

- You may feel that love is a dangerous and unsafe war zone.
- You may struggle to believe you're worthy of love, or you may be waiting for your partner to become hurtful.
- You may desperately want love.
- You may struggle with boundaries or have extra awareness of boundaries.

TYPE OF ATTACHMENTS

AVOIDANT

This is believed to be formed by having your needs rejected or diminished as an infant—the child learns not to ask for comfort as they feel they won't be responded to.

- You may find sharing feelings uncomfortable.
- You might have problems with intimacy and commitment.
- You might feel smothered in relationships.
- You may fear losing your independence.
- You may be independent and capable.
- People may call you "cold" or "heartless."

SECURE

This is believed to be formed by getting most of your needs met as an infant.

- You are generally comfortable depending on others and having others depend on you.
- Communicating your feelings feels relatively easy.
- You don't fear being abandoned or cheated on.
- You don't fear others getting too close.
- You can set boundaries in relationships.
- You don't need a romantic relationship to feel complete.

ANXIOUS

These people may call or text a lot, be jealous, manipulate others to get some kind of reaction, ignore red flags so that they can still be in a relationship, or people-please.

DISORGANIZED

These people may exhibit both anxious and avoidant characteristics—pulling away from people who want to get close, yet feeling anxious with avoidant people.

BEHAVIOR IN RELATIONSHIPS

AVOIDANT

These people may ghost or break off relationships, long for the phantom ex (even while in a new relationship), set extremely high expectations, or magnify their partner's flaws.

SECURE

These people can examine themselves, communicate their needs, express boundaries, are honest with their feelings, and will tell their partner what they're feeling, instead of wishing the partner to simply know.

Our attachment style can also change and be affected by other key relationships and significant events. A particularly good and impactful friendship can make us more trusting, whereas being cheated on can make us more anxious. It is situational and depends on the individual, too.

There can be some shaming and demonizing of certain attachment styles—especially avoidant types, who are often labeled as cold—but remember that all of them are equally valid. It is perfectly okay to desire more space or more closeness in your relationships, but we can work with partners to ease insecurity and lessen our own extreme behaviors.

WHAT MAKES A RELATIONSHIP TOXIC OR ABUSIVE?

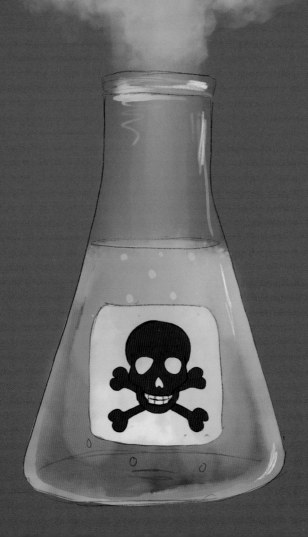

The more awareness of abuse and the different forms it can take, and what it can look like, the better. Each year in the United States, an estimated 10 million people experience domestic violence. **More than one in three women and one in four men in the US will experience rape, physical violence, and/or stalking by an intimate partner.**

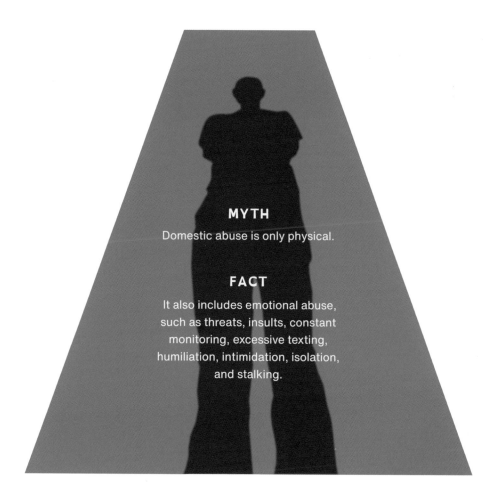

MYTH
Domestic abuse is only physical.

FACT

It also includes emotional abuse, such as threats, insults, constant monitoring, excessive texting, humiliation, intimidation, isolation, and stalking.

RED FLAGS

Abusive relationships often start with smaller things that you brush off, or that could feel exciting in the beginning. While the following are not all signs that someone will become abusive, they are points to be aware of:

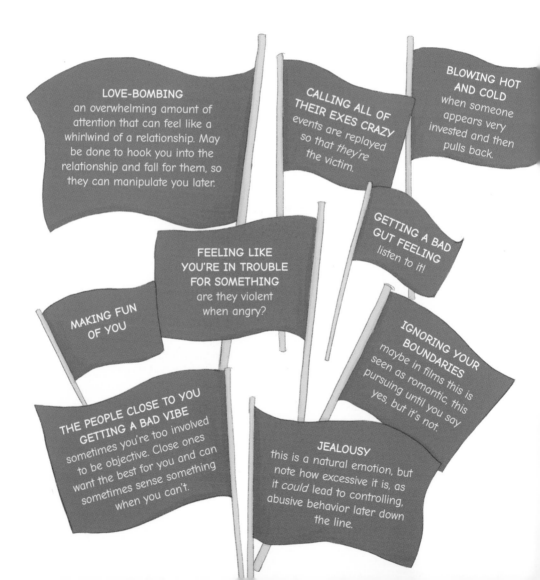

LOVE-BOMBING
an overwhelming amount of attention that can feel like a whirlwind of a relationship. May be done to hook you into the relationship and fall for them, so they can manipulate you later.

CALLING ALL OF THEIR EXES CRAZY
events are replayed so that they're the victim.

BLOWING HOT AND COLD
when someone appears very invested and then pulls back.

GETTING A BAD GUT FEELING
listen to it!

FEELING LIKE YOU'RE IN TROUBLE FOR SOMETHING
are they violent when angry?

MAKING FUN OF YOU

IGNORING YOUR BOUNDARIES
maybe in films this is seen as romantic, this pursuing until you say yes, but it's not.

THE PEOPLE CLOSE TO YOU GETTING A BAD VIBE
sometimes you're too involved to be objective. Close ones want the best for you and can sometimes sense something when you can't.

JEALOUSY
this is a natural emotion, but note how excessive it is, as it could lead to controlling, abusive behavior later down the line.

GREEN FLAGS

If you're used to explosive, rocky relationships, when you experience a healthier one, it may feel a bit boring as you're not used to it, and it may take time to adjust. Don't sabotage a relationship because it doesn't feel dramatic, obsessive, or unpredictable.

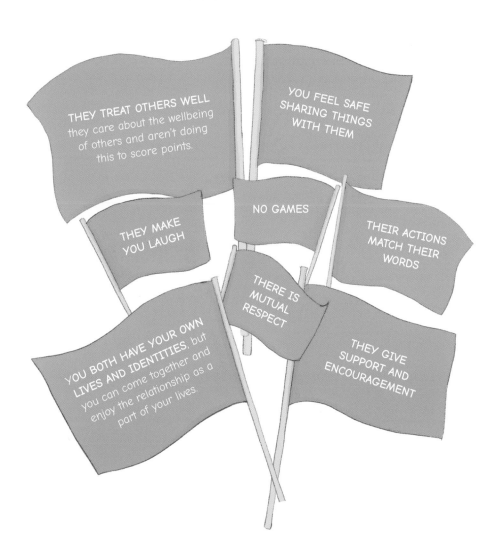

THEY TREAT OTHERS WELL
they care about the wellbeing of others and aren't doing this to score points.

YOU FEEL SAFE SHARING THINGS WITH THEM

THEY MAKE YOU LAUGH

NO GAMES

THEIR ACTIONS MATCH THEIR WORDS

YOU BOTH HAVE YOUR OWN LIVES AND IDENTITIES, but you can come together and enjoy the relationship as a part of your lives.

THERE IS MUTUAL RESPECT

THEY GIVE SUPPORT AND ENCOURAGEMENT

ARGUMENTS + CONFLICT MANAGEMENT

While arguments are very natural, and even necessary in a relationship, we're not very good at arguing. Our egos get in the way and we can feel attacked, so rather than showing our vulnerability and pain, it may feel easier to be combative. The psychologist Dr. John Gottman identified what he named the Four Horsemen of the Apocalypse—common relationship problems that can presage the end of a relationship. But he also offers up antidotes:

STONEWALLING
when someone withdraws completely from the conversation. The antidote is to take a break for twenty minutes to get out of the heated moment, to think and take pause, and then return to talk.

DEFENSIVENESS
protecting yourself, sometimes through denial and playing the victim. The antidote is to recognize and accept some of the responsibility.

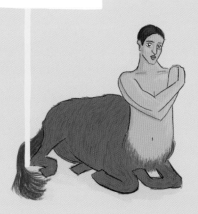

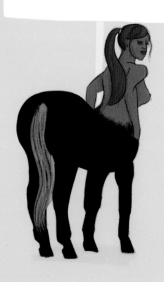

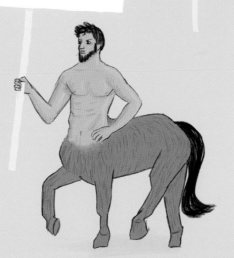

CRITICISM
constantly attacking your partner's character as opposed to the problem in hand. The antidote is saying "I" instead of "you," as it can feel less personal to your partner.

CONTEMPT
an air of superiority cast over your partner through sarcasm, mockery, eye-rolling, or cynicism. The antidote is to be respectful and appreciative, and to meet on a more equal playing field.

Arguments can be constructive and reveal things that have been brewing and haven't been said. They can form the path back to connection—if our egos don't get in the way.

BOUNDARIES

Sometimes saying yes might feel like the kindest thing when you want to avoid confrontation. But poor boundaries can lead to anger or resentment further down the line, and are more likely to be violated if you hold them in and don't communicate them.

HOW TO SET BOUNDARIES

You're allowed to have boundaries! It's not an unkind thing, but have some patience while first navigating them as people aren't perfect. Setting boundaries can sound like:

MENTAL BOUNDARY
"We think differently and I respect your opinion, but please don't force it on me."

TIME BOUNDARY
"I can only stay for an hour," or "If you're going to be late, please let me know ahead of time," or "I'll respond to all work emails first thing in the morning."

MATERIAL BOUNDARY
"Please ask me first if you'd like to use my . . ."

EMOTIONAL DUMPING BOUNDARY
"I want to be there for you, but I am unable to support you in the way you need right now."

THE CYCLE OF ABUSE

The psychologist Lenore Walker theorized that abuse usually takes on a cyclical nature, which reinforces how difficult it is to leave.

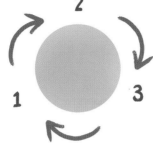

ACUTE VIOLENCE
violence erupts

2

TENSION-BUILDING PHASE
a gradual escalation of aggression

1

3

HONEYMOON PHASE
the abusive partner may apologize, give gifts, show remorse, and make false promises, to convince that it won't happen again

MYTH

If the abuse was bad enough, they'd leave.

FACT

Relationships are rarely violent from the start. There was initially a foundation of love that was built. Once you are in that web, it can be hard to escape, especially if finances/children are involved; your safety is threatened if you leave; manipulation is used to persuade you that they'll change; they gaslight you. There are so many reasons why it's not easy to leave.

LIVING WITH VIOLENCE

The Women's Aid Federation recommends making a plan to increase your safety:

- Plan responses to different scenarios.
- Plan who you could go to in an emergency.
- Pack an emergency bag.
- Carry a little money at all times, for buses or trains.

- If you think a partner is going to attack you, is there a room that is lower risk? Avoid the kitchen with its knives, or places where you could be cornered with no escape.

EMERGENCY BAG

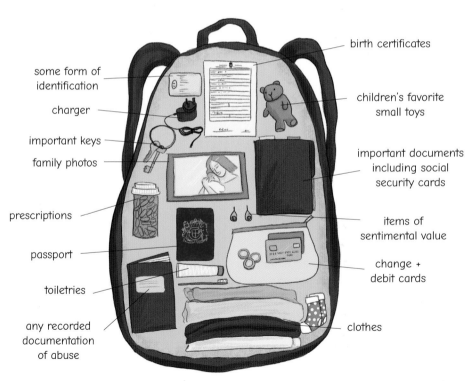

- some form of identification
- charger
- important keys
- family photos
- prescriptions
- passport
- toiletries
- any recorded documentation of abuse

- birth certificates
- children's favorite small toys
- important documents including social security cards
- items of sentimental value
- change + debit cards
- clothes

ASK FOR HELP

If you need support in leaving an abusive situation, the National Domestic Violence Hotline (thehotline.org) can be reached by call, text, or chat. They can help you leave, connect you with local resources, and plan a path to safety.

If you are feeling unsafe while out at a bar or on a date, communicate in code and ask the bartender for an "angel shot" to let them know that you are in need of assistance.

LEAVING VIOLENCE

This can be a dangerous time, so if you're able to, plan with care:

- Inform family, work, and your children's school of the situation and ask them not to give your address or telephone number to anyone.
- Try to alter your regular routes, places, and appointments, where your partner knows to look for you.
- If possible, avoid using shared bank accounts.

- Be aware that voting is a matter of public record in the US and can help an abuser determine your location.

For more comprehensive advice on dealing with abusive relationships, see the Further Reading on page 212.

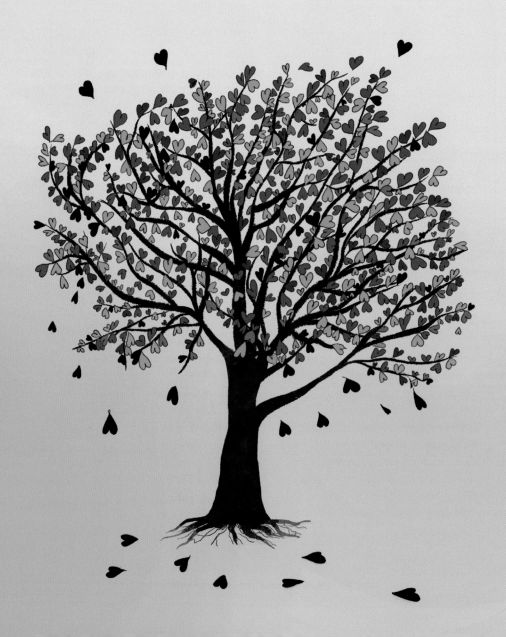

When we start a new relationship, we try not to imagine its ending—we're just exploring and getting to know someone new. Yet endings happen and can be as tricky to initiate as to deal with. But let's try. (*Note*: this advice relates to fully consensual relationships; see page 15 for reflections on toxic and abusive relationships.)

HOW TO BREAK UP WITH SOMEONE

- Be sure this is what you want to do, after some consideration, and that there is nothing that can be worked through together or by means of a conversation.
- Be honest, yet sensitive to the other person's feelings.
- Apologize and explain (thank them for everything, if appropriate).
- Be prepared for them not to take it well.
- Consider the other person's feelings when you're deciding where to break up.
- Try to avoid doing it in the heat of an argument, when you may say things that you regret later on, and which might tarnish the whole relationship with that last memory.
- Don't leave things open-ended, as this can make it harder for you both to move on and get over the breakup.

While nothing will particularly help with the immediate pain that you may both feel, there are some actions that will definitely make things worse for the other party:

- **Cheating** as a way of avoiding the difficult conversation, or to get the other person to end the relationship.
- **Using a special occasion** (e.g., their birthday) to break up.
- **Ghosting** (different from drifting apart) is when someone has decided it's easier to cut off communication than to have a difficult conversation. It can be hurtful to the other party as they have been left with no explanation as to what happened; a relationship that they thought was valuable seemingly wasn't so to you.

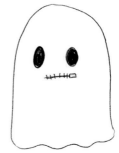

HOW TO DEAL WITH A BREAKUP

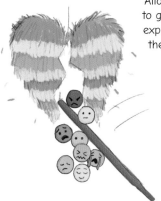

Allow yourself to grieve or to experience all the feelings.

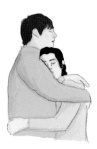

Surround yourself by other comforting things and people; talk it through and confide in others.

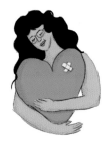

Try to build self-esteem from within (see page 11) and from others who love you, rather than relying on getting worth solely through starting new relationships straight after a breakup.

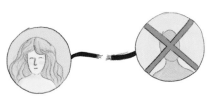

If you're not over your ex, or had a bad experience with them, try blocking them on social media until your feelings are more muted. It may help to distance yourself from the relationship.

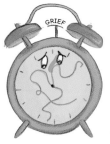

Avoid the narrative "I *should* be over it by now"— everyone grieves differently and it could take anywhere from days to years to heal.

GRIEVING A FRIENDSHIP BREAKUP

We expect so much from our romantic relationships, and if something doesn't work, we break up and move on to the next. With friendships, there's often less pressure for one friend to meet quite as many needs. Yet we all experience friendship endings and stalemates, which can be just as painful.

We don't tend to have the same expectations of friendships that we have of romantic relationships—perhaps because if we only see friends every now and then, we don't want to ruin that quality time. However, this can lead to two people being on different pages about the friendship. Somehow, with a romance ending, there's hope of finding another one: there are tales of new loves and plenty of advice on how to rediscover yourself after a breakup. Yet each friendship is unique and offers something different, so it can be difficult to replicate that same relationship—for instance, it's impossible to replace a childhood friend who knew you when you were young. Different friends bring out different facets of your personality and interests.

Friendships are often brittle at times of change: moving away, changing jobs, starting a family, and so on. With each change come more life obstacles and less time to invest in old friendships; that shines a light on whether you want to keep investing time in that friendship.

Perhaps a friendship naturally fizzled out and both of you stopped making an effort; maybe an explosive argument occurred; or one friend changed and the other didn't; perhaps they ghosted you—whatever the reason, absent friends can still leave a big void, along with the memories, some of which you may look back on in a grateful, warming way when they enter your mind, and others not so much. Not every friend and partner will be lifelong, and that's okay! As with other things, the duration of a relationship doesn't equate to its value.

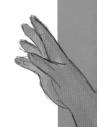

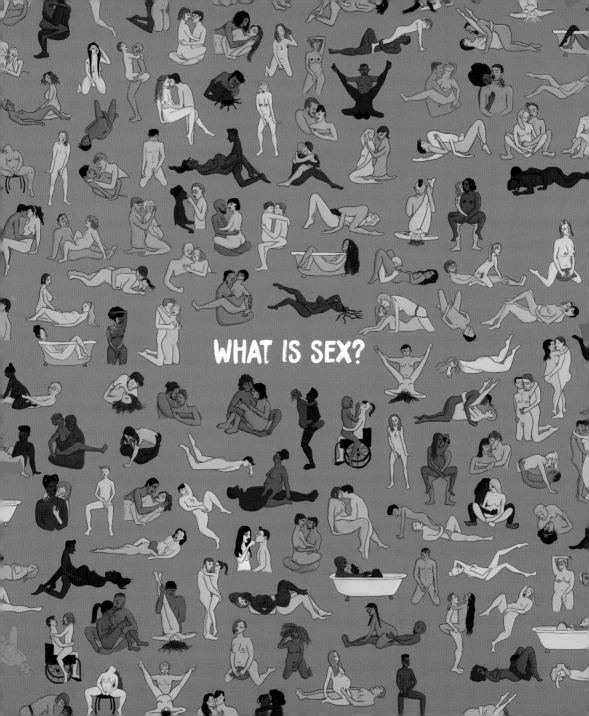

WHAT IS SEX?

Mammals have been reproducing for hundreds of millions of years (fossilized remains revealed the first embryo and umbilical cord were found inside the soon-to-be mother's body 380 million years ago). But as our civilizations have formed and evolved, attitudes towards sex have changed, too. Fast forward to today: something natural and necessary for all animals has become something that humans have grown ashamed of, something not to discuss in polite society.

It's important to look at how attitudes towards the purpose of sex developed—oscillating between procreation and pleasure. Sex that isn't solely for procreation opens up what the definition of sex can encompass—no longer only penis-in-vagina sex, no longer a sole focus on male ejaculation, no longer only heterocentric sex. We can unpick sex education from a sex-negative society and question our own shame about sexuality (if we haven't already).

WHY IS SEX SO TABOO?

Where sexual shame in the Western world originated is much debated. One traceable link could be to Plato (c.427–347 BCE), who spearheaded the concept of the untainted soul vs. the soiled body, and the idea that only sacred love resulted in true happiness. Therefore, physical love and sexual desire were seen as regressing humans to an animal state, rather than aspiring to acquire higher immaterial spirituality.

There are many examples of sexual shame throughout cultures, both historically and today, especially around suppressing female pleasure and homosexual pleasure. With female pleasure specifically, shame most probably evolved with the rise in agriculture. When agriculture replaced the tribal sharing of land, tasks, food, and parenting, there was a need to ascertain which baby belonged to which father, in order to pass down their segment of land and assets to their bloodline. Enter . . . the patriarchy, which controlled women, commoditized them, and limited their sexuality, valuing virginity and resulting in slut-shaming! For men, sex was meant to be some sort of conquest, with domination and virility at the center, leaving little room for those who don't particularly want that sort of sex.

VIRGINITY

The fascination with virginity has been around for millennia, again dating back to the rise in agriculture around 12,000 years ago. The forming of patriarchal societies resulted in fathers being able to sell their daughters as pregnancy vessels—the cultural reinforcement of the importance of virginity, and monogamous marriages, would give the groom peace of mind that there was no possibility of his wife's pregnancy with another man's child.

This fixation led to the creation of countless virginity tests throughout history. However, a 2017 systemic review of virginity testing found that virginity examination is not a useful clinical tool and can be physically, socially, and psychologically devastating to the examinees. From a human-rights perspective, virginity testing is a form of gender discrimination as well as a violation of fundamental rights and, when carried out without consent, a form of sexual assault. Such virginity tests have led to devastating, unnecessary consequences and punishment for women all over the world.

VIRGINITY TEST MYTHS

BLOOD ON SHEETS

= VIRGIN

CARRYING WATER IN A SIEVE

= VIRGIN

SPARKLING URINE

= VIRGIN

TAMING A UNICORN

IF 2 FINGERS FIT IN VAGINA

= NOT VIRGIN

BOOBS THAT POINT DOWNWARDS

= NOT VIRGIN

= VIRGIN

MYTH

The hymen remains "intact" before penetrative sex.

FACT

The hymen starts as one unbroken structure at birth, but by puberty it should have worn into more of a ring of tissue— the vaginal corona, which also lets out menstrual blood. There is such a thing as an imperforate hymen, which requires a procedure to create the hole. However, generally the membrane won't cover the entire vagina, there's nothing to be "popped," and you cannot tell whether or not someone has had sex by looking at their vagina!

SEX IS SO MUCH MORE THAN PIV

SENSUAL BATH

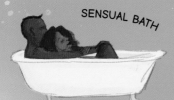

EXPLORING EROGENOUS ZONES

KISSING SESH

LUST

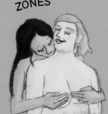

FUN WITH FOOD

SEXTING

EROTIC

WATCHING PORN TOGETHER

SOLO PLAY

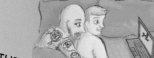

GIVE EACH OTHER A HAND

SEXY DANCING

ROLE PLAY

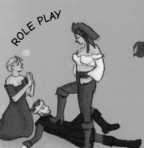

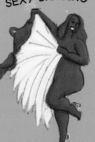

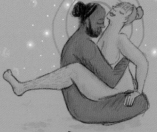

TANTRIC SEX

BUTT FUN

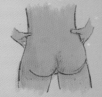

EROTIC ASMR

TEMPERATURE PLAY

KINK

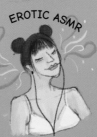

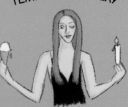

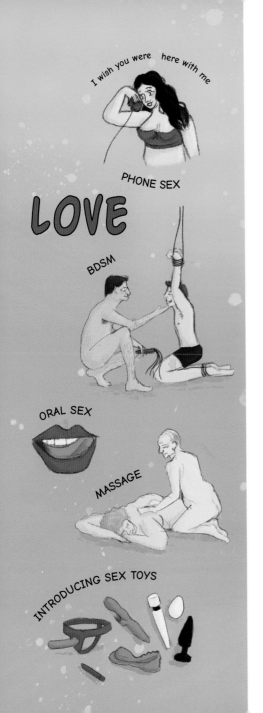

I wish you were here with me

PHONE SEX

LOVE

BDSM

ORAL SEX

MASSAGE

INTRODUCING SEX TOYS

HOW DO YOU DEFINE SEX?

When I grew up, school gossip revolved around metaphorical baseball bases:

1ST BASE
= kissing and fondling

2ND BASE
= fingering/hand job

3RD BASE
= oral sex

4TH BASE
= penetrative sex
(the "ultimate goal")

What a narrow script of what sex can be! It excludes many people who don't want, or can't have, that kind of sex, and is very much based on a heteronormative view of what type of sex is "normal." Sex can be a whole world of fun, and PIV sex may be a small part of that or not a part of it at all. There is a whole menu of items, so that everyone involved can still have a great time.

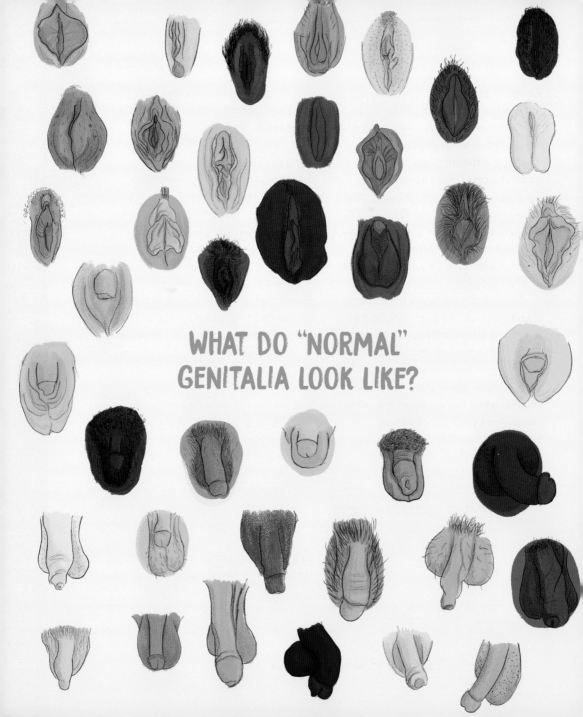

WHAT DO "NORMAL" GENITALIA LOOK LIKE?

GET TO KNOW YOURSELF

We rarely get to see other vulvas and penises in the flesh, so it's natural to wonder what is normal. Well, genitalia are as unique as fingerprints, and they're all different in shape, size, and color. The only points of reference you may have had when growing up are textbooks where you see a single diagram; some of your sexual partners; or mainstream porn, where penises are large and hard, vulvas are neat and tucked, and pubes are often mythical.

If you have a vulva, it's hard to see it, and we're encouraged to treat it as something taboo and not to be talked about. We're not even taught the correct terminology: "vulva" and "vagina" often get confused. Many still use the word "vagina" when talking about the vulva. The author Lynn Enright argues that "It's still such a taboo to say 'vulva' as we don't like to talk about female genitalia except in relation to male sexuality. The vagina is something that a penis can

go into, and a baby can come out of, so we've become more comfortable with that word."

With female pleasure in particular being such a taboo, it's common for many people to have never actually looked at their own vulvas.

With little discussion or reference on offer, no wonder there is a lot of insecurity and dissatisfaction concerning one's own vulva.

Take a look at yours and get acquainted, and have a peek in the Further Reading section (page 212) for more examples, to discover the diversity of genitalia out there.

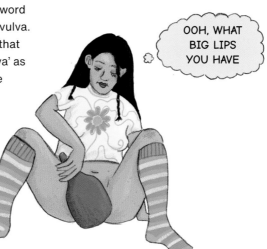

OOH, WHAT
BIG LIPS
YOU HAVE

THE VULVA

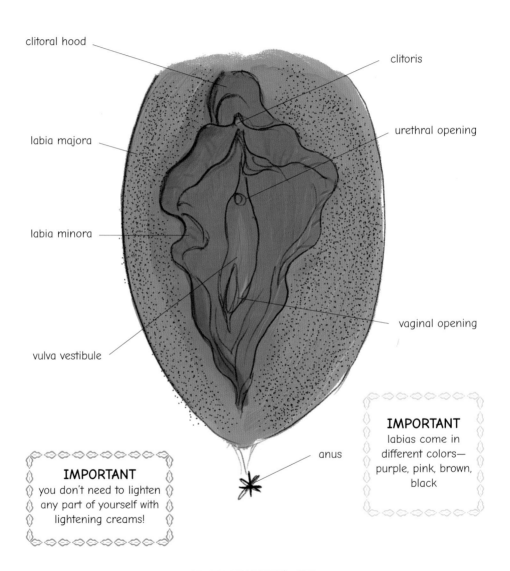

clitoral hood

clitoris

labia majora

urethral opening

labia minora

vulva vestibule

vaginal opening

anus

DISTINCT ODORS

The vagina is not meant to smell like fresh berries! It has its own smell, which may be coppery, musky, or fleshy. "Feminine hygiene" washes are not needed and can disrupt the vaginal microbiome, an ecosystem of microbes, bacteria, and fungi in the vagina that helps protect against pathogens, fight off yeast infections, and perform other miracles. Mild soap for washing your vulva works just fine, and the vagina itself is a self-cleaning machine!

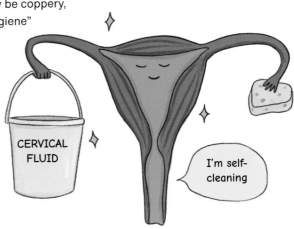

CERVICAL FLUID

I'm self-cleaning

VAGINAL pH

The vagina is acidic (with a pH level of between 3.8 and 4.5) in order to keep itself clean, so if you notice slightly orange stains in your underwear, this is why.

INTERSEX

This is the general term for people whose genitalia don't fit the typical categories of male or female. Different doctors and medical professionals have different views on what counts as intersex, and it doesn't neatly fit into any one category. A person might have "mosaic genetics"—some chromosomes that are XX and some that are XY—or "ambiguous genitalia."

DISCHARGE: WHAT IS IT?

Vaginal discharge is normal and healthy, and encompasses cervical fluid and vaginal lubrication. Cervical fluid/mucus—produced by the cervix—aids in getting pregnant, cleans the vagina, and protects from infection.

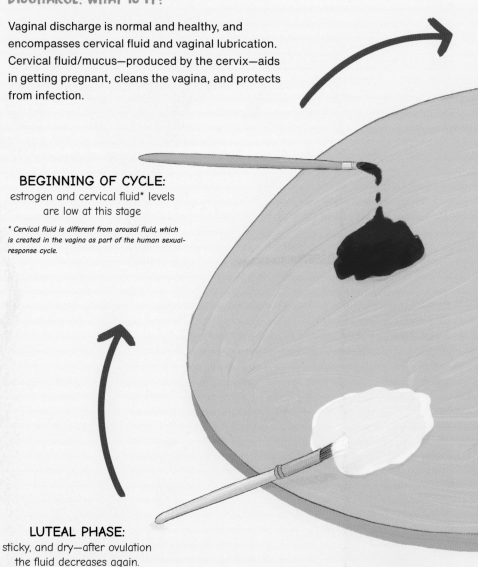

BEGINNING OF CYCLE:
estrogen and cervical fluid* levels
are low at this stage

*Cervical fluid is different from arousal fluid, which is created in the vagina as part of the human sexual-response cycle.

LUTEAL PHASE:
sticky, and dry—after ovulation
the fluid decreases again.

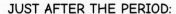

JUST AFTER THE PERIOD:
absent, dry, cloudy, and white/yellow
as estrogen levels rise slowly.

LEAD-UP TO OVULATION:
sticky, white, creamy, and lotion-y
as estrogen levels rise more and
the cervix produces more fluid.
It can be sticky or tacky to begin
with, then become wetter
and creamier.

BACTERIAL VAGINOSIS
discharge that is gray in colour is
most commonly a sign of BV.

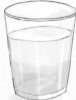

AROUND OVULATION:
thin, slippery, wet, clear,
with the consistency of
egg whites—fluid becomes
wetter and slippery, then
stretchy and clear.

STIs
green discharge could be a sign of a
bacterial infection or an STI.

ARE YOU A GROWER OR A SHOW-ER?

There is also no correlation between the size of a penis when it's flaccid and when it's fully erect. Some are small and remain small; some are small and get bigger; some are big and harden; some are big and grow even more. All are completely normal!

PENIS SIZE

You may have heard the saying "You can tell the size of a penis by the size of someone's feet." It's a myth, debunked by a 2002 study by the *British Journal of Urology*, which showed that there is no statistically significant correlation between shoe size and stretched penis length.

UNCIRCUMCISED PENIS

Uncircumcised penises aren't less hygienic—they just need to be washed under the foreskin.

WET DREAMS

All genders can have them. While more common in puberty, they can also happen into adulthood.

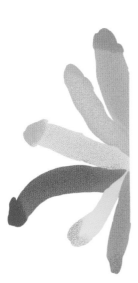

THE ANGLE OF THE DANGLE

Erections can be upright, point down, stick out at a 90-degree angle, or anywhere in between, and having a slight curve in the penis is considered normal, too. While a little curve can be normal, an extreme bend may be a sign of Peyronie's disease.

ERECTILE DYSFUNCTION (ED)

This doesn't necessarily mean that you're not attracted to your partner: there are many things that cause it, including stress, lifestyle, health problems, and medication.

NOCTURNAL PENILE TUMESCENCE

Did you know that regular nighttime erections—a.k.a. nocturnal penile tumescence—are a sign that your body is in good health? You may get them three to five times per night. If you have ED but you can regularly get erections throughout the night, this is a sign that it's a psychological issue, not a physiological one.

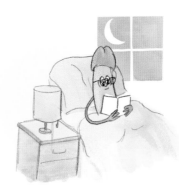

WHAT IS THE CLITORIS?

The clitoris has eluded us for thousands of years. Whether
that's because there's a dispiriting lack of research
into female pleasure, or because certain scientists and
psychologists spread misinformation (Freud, I'm looking
at you),* or a combination of the two, the shocking fact is
that the first images of the clitoral structure surfaced only
in 1998, thanks to the urologist Dr. Helen O'Connell. Rather
than being just the little nub you can see externally, the
clitoris is in fact much more integral and forms the basis
of all female orgasms.

*Freud believed that clitoral orgasms were immature—a result of penis envy—and
that only vaginal orgasm was mature and healthy.*

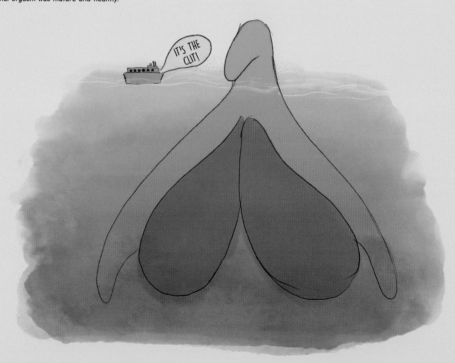

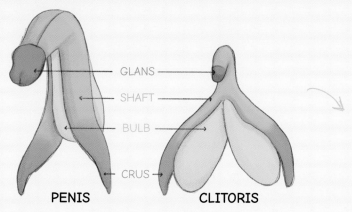

GLANS

SHAFT

BULB

CRUS

PENIS   **CLITORIS**

The penis and clitoris are homologous structures.

G SPOT MYTHOLOGY

There is no physical evidence of the G spot. A study proposed instead a clitourethrovaginal complex, based on anatomical relationships between the clitoris, the urethra, and the anterior vaginal wall that could, when properly stimulated, induce orgasm. The clitoris is very similar in structure to the male sexual organs—it contains lots of nerves, so it can be super-sensitive.

THE ORGASM GAP

A study in 2017 highlighted an issue called the "orgasm gap" by exploring orgasm rates between heterosexual men, heterosexual women, gay men, bisexual men, bisexual women, and lesbians.

People of all genders orgasmed 95 percent of the time when engaging in solo play. When with a partner, heterosexual men said they usually always orgasmed, remaining at 95 percent, with gay men (89 percent), bisexual men (88 percent), and lesbians (86 percent) coming in fairly close behind. However, bisexual and heterosexual women get a raw deal, orgasming only 65 percent of the time. From this, we can see that the issue is not a biological one, but a social one.

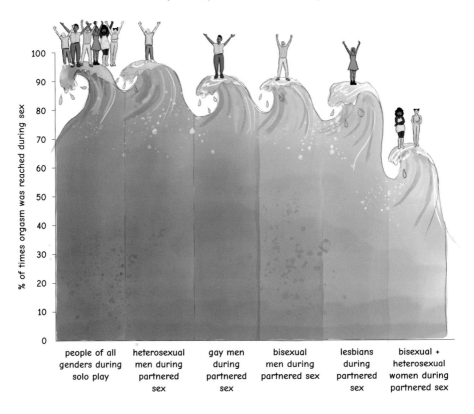

But why? Many reasons come into play:

1. **The personal is political:** years of inequality in general have undoubtedly had a domino effect in the bedroom. Men have historically enjoyed various privileges and basic rights that women could not, so of course orgasm inequality in heterosexual relationships is there as well. Perhaps male ejaculate being needed for procreation made society more accepting of male orgasms. While people have banded together in the streets and advocated loudly for societal equality, between the sheets it can end up being a solo mission between you and your partner.

2. **Sex myths:** some myths about sex and female anatomy are believed and internalized—for example, female pleasure being too complex or taking too long.

3. **Mindset:** this can lead heterosexual cis men in particular to not try, and to women who sleep with men worrying that they're taking too long and that their pleasure is a nuisance, which doesn't create an encouraging atmosphere for orgasms. If partners start with the expectation that the man will climax and the woman may or may not, that may determine the sequence of events and the outcome of the encounter.

The contemporary phrase "Don't give me blue balls" (referring to discomfort caused through arousal not ending in orgasm) and the more historical—and no less horrifying—"Close your eyes and think of England" (meaning "don't refuse a man's sexual advances") demonstrate this dark entitlement to an orgasm presiding over a woman's right to consent. For most of modern history, sex was seen as something a woman had to endure rather than enjoy—but no longer.

OOOH!

MYTH

Only testicles can experience pain from prolonged arousal without orgasm.

FACT

Vulvas can experience the same pain. The discomfort/pain for both sexes can be relieved by orgasm, but partners should not be coerced into having sex in order to provide it. Just masturbate alone if your partner doesn't want to continue.

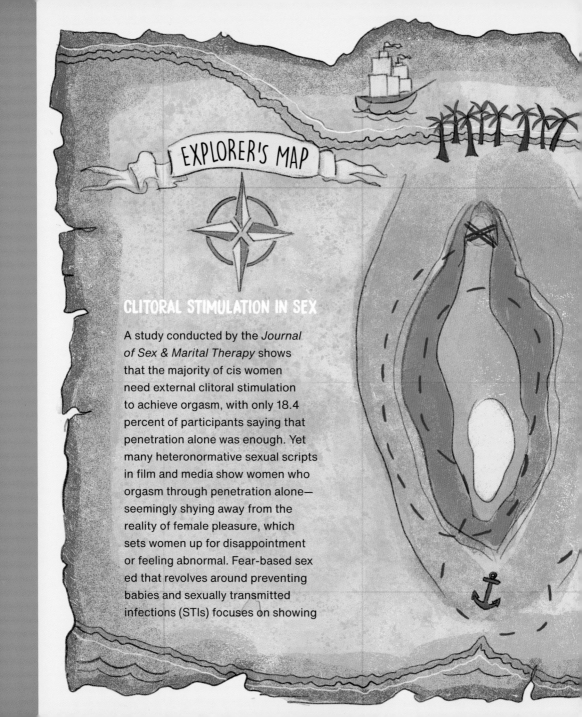

CLITORAL STIMULATION IN SEX

A study conducted by the *Journal of Sex & Marital Therapy* shows that the majority of cis women need external clitoral stimulation to achieve orgasm, with only 18.4 percent of participants saying that penetration alone was enough. Yet many heteronormative sexual scripts in film and media show women who orgasm through penetration alone—seemingly shying away from the reality of female pleasure, which sets women up for disappointment or feeling abnormal. Fear-based sex ed that revolves around preventing babies and sexually transmitted infections (STIs) focuses on showing how to use a condom and disposing of it after ejaculation; this education implies that the male orgasm is a given, and the female orgasm is an insignificant partner to the main attraction. See also the "money shot" in mainstream porn, where the male performer ejaculates and the scene is over.

The study also explored what type of stimulation cis women enjoy receiving, and the results showed "considerable diversity in genital touch preferences," with some women preferring 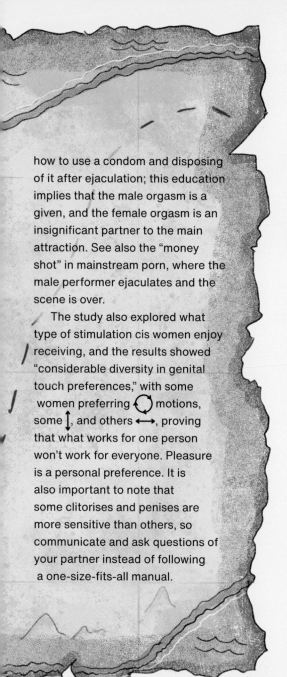 motions, some ↕, and others ↔, proving that what works for one person won't work for everyone. Pleasure is a personal preference. It is also important to note that some clitorises and penises are more sensitive than others, so communicate and ask questions of your partner instead of following a one-size-fits-all manual.

LET'S TALK MALE PLEASURE

While female pleasure is taboo, so in a way is male pleasure. In bro culture, when discussing sexual exploits and masturbation, most men don't talk about sensations and the emotions felt; language instead focuses on pounding and how long you lasted. Pleasure itself seems taboo. Perhaps that has to do with the fact that men aren't encouraged to express their emotions as much as women.

This seems to have had a domino effect on the sex toy market. While the sex toy market is booming, the majority of toys are marketed for women. Yet male sex toys are available—and they are there for pleasure!

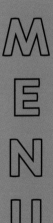
CLITORAL

....

Vibrators can be buzzy or rumbling—ask your server to give you a sample of both to see which you prefer. Test on the tip of your nose to see what your cup of tea is.

Bullet
Great place to start

Pebble

Novelty

Suction
Emulates blowing/
sucking sensation

Wider surface area

Wearable
Can turn finger into
vibrator

Hands free
Tuck behind labia
folds

PENILE

....

**Masturbation
sleeve**

Stroker

Cock ring

VAGINAL

....

Thruster

Dildo
Explore different
materials, such as glass
or metal, for different
sensations

Rabbit
Dual function. Penetrative
with clitoral stimulation

ANAL

Anal beads

Beads increase in size, offering options

Butt plugs

Best to start small and work your way up.

Dildo

All come with a flared base as the anus is surprisingly vacuum-like

OTHERS

Prostate massager

Grind-on toy

For the grinders of the world

Wand vibrator

Originally invented to soothe sore muscles, this toy offers an intense experience. Not for the faint-hearted

SIDES

Lube
recommended with any choice of toy to enhance the experience!

Condoms
use with toys if they're being shared to help prevent STIs

SPECIALS

SERVES 2

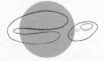

Remote-controlled

BDSM play

To be used in conjunction with safe words, and extra care

Handcuffs

App-controlled

A revolutionary invention, perfect for long-distance relationships

Strap-on

WHAT IS GOOD SEX?

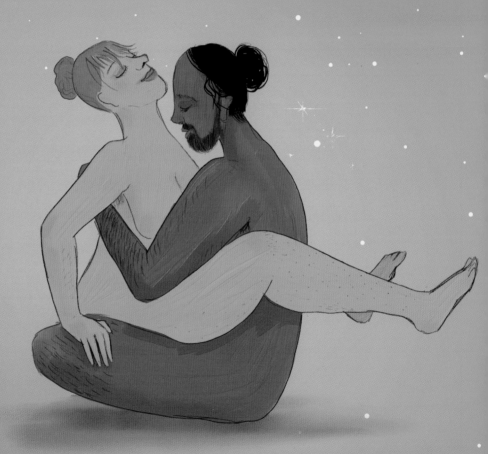

There is something so vulnerable about sex. And the perception of what "good" and "bad" sex looks like gets wrapped up in our egos and our expectations of others. Sex is seemingly everywhere, yet we're also brought up in a society that is fairly awkward and shies away from it, with many people being left to figure things out on their own. While there are initiatives to improve sex education, unfortunately not everyone gets the in-depth sex ed they deserve. This gap can lead to bad sex when education comes in the form of cultural myths, mainstream porn, and tales from bragging friends and magazines. Generalist advice on specific sex techniques should be taken with a grain of salt, as what works for one person might not work for someone else! Ask your partner what they like, and try things out together that you both like the sound of. Sex is something that is learned through experience and practice. It doesn't always have to be perfect!

Many youngsters have porn as their introduction to sex, but don't get the education around it. As I learned from ethical porn performers and producers King Noire and Jet Setting Jasmine in a talk they gave on the subject, there is plenty that goes on behind the scenes that we don't witness: porn performers train to be able to do these contortionist positions, there are big vats of lube you don't see, and porn is created with entertainment in mind. Porn can give inspiration, but using mainstream porn as the sole how-to guide for sex can create some unrealistic expectations of partners in the bedroom.

There's a lot of pressure concerning what we should be doing and experiencing, as well as how we should look and sound, during sex. Yet this leaves out how sex can be much more complicated, funny, emotional, and unique than that.

AS A RULE
OF THUMB,
SEX SHOULD BE:

CONSENSUAL

SAFE

PLEASURABLE
for everyone involved

Beyond that, it can be many things—the rest is up to you.

THINGS YOU DON'T SEE IN MAINSTREAM PORN

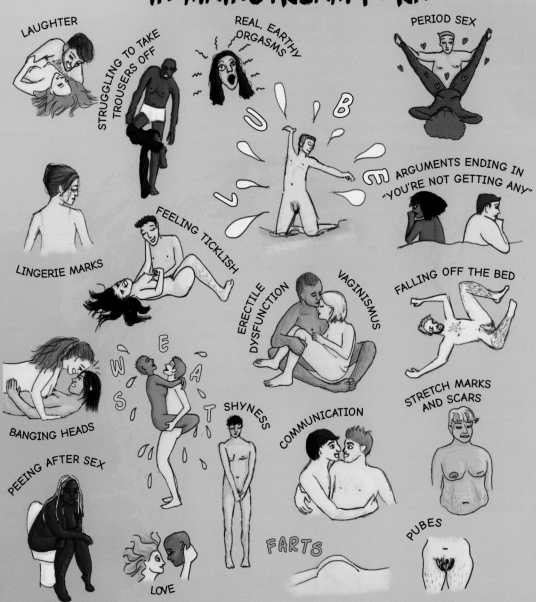

LAUGHTER

STRUGGLING TO TAKE TROUSERS OFF

REAL, EARTHY ORGASMS

PERIOD SEX

ARGUMENTS ENDING IN "YOU'RE NOT GETTING ANY"

LINGERIE MARKS

FEELING TICKLISH

ERECTILE DYSFUNCTION

VAGINISMUS

FALLING OFF THE BED

BANGING HEADS

SHYNESS

COMMUNICATION

STRETCH MARKS AND SCARS

PEEING AFTER SEX

LOVE

FARTS

PUBES

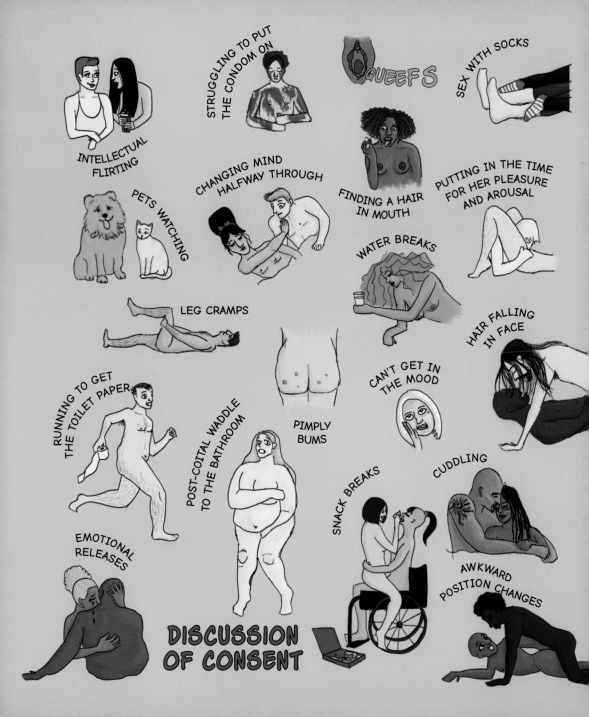

HOW DOES DESIRE WORK, AND HOW DO I MAINTAIN IT?

To get a better sense of how desire works, I spoke to Dr. Karen Gurney (a.k.a., the Sex Doctor), who is a clinical psychologist and psychosexologist and the author of *Mind the Gap: The Truth About Desire and How to Futureproof Your Sex Life.* Karen works at 56 Dean Street, Europe's busiest sexual health, contraception, and HIV care clinic, located in the heart of London's Soho (the medical center was once called the "The Beyoncé of Sexual Health Clinics").

We explored how to cultivate desire within existing relationships and find both comfort and novelty in a relationship. Here are some of Karen's reflections on what we tend to get wrong about sex, arousal, and desire, as well as some clinically backed recommendations for keeping the flame alive.

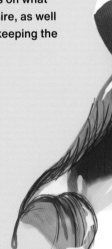

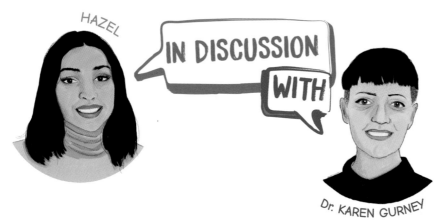

HAZEL

IN DISCUSSION WITH

Dr. KAREN GURNEY

Why does desire dwindle the longer people have been together? Is it normal? Is it inevitable? What should we know?

One of the things that we know from sex research is that people tend to experience higher levels of spontaneous desire at the beginning of a relationship because their partner is novel. And our brains really like novel sexual stimuli—something we've not seen or done before is quite exciting to us. Over time in these relationship dynamics, the other person gets really well known to us. That almost kind of dilutes them as a sexual being, and we start having relationships with them other than a sexual one: so we become good friends, we might be roommates if we live together, we might become co-parents.

There are things that we might find irritating, or things that are just quite predictable, including things like how they initiate sex. It might seem that it would be easier to have more sex, because you live together. But actually we know that when people cohabit, they tend to have a bit less sex. That's because if the opportunity is always there, you might just put it off for tomorrow. You don't have the [positive] trigger that a date night might bring. Thinking about the date, getting ready for the date, thinking about what might happen are really good triggers for desire, which you miss out on if you're living together.

How can you rekindle the spark in a relationship?

The first thing is understanding how desire works: the way in which we've been sold an idea of desire—something that is natural, and we should just feel—is wrong. Desire is something that often needs nurturing and triggering. When we sit around waiting for desire to happen, it often doesn't. And we know sex isn't a drive, because the less we have, the less we crave. Most people feel that when they're not feeling like sex, there's something wrong with them or there's something wrong with their relationship. And that's not the case.

The thing I think makes the most difference is to increase what I call "sexual currency"—it's the charge between you and another person. It's flirting, it's physical affection that's a bit more sexual; it might be texts that are suggestive, it might be compliments about how much you're attracted to that person, it might be being naked together, it might be sexual touch, physical touch that's more sexual, but isn't necessarily something you'd call sex.

There's this idea that our sexuality is either off or it's on. Actually, our sexuality—both alone and in our relationship—is something that can always be around if we want it to be, in the way that we are, in the way that we think, in the way that we dress, in the way that we dance, in the way that we touch each other, in the way that we kiss when we say goodbye, in the way in which we write texts. And all of those things provide a scaffolding to help people move easily from a non-sexual place, like taking the trash out together, to more of a sexual place, without awkwardness, and with the trigger for desire.

Where it usually goes wrong is when people allow that sexual currency to deplete over time. Passionate kissing outside of sex, for example, is something that people find themselves doing less and less, but it's exactly that passionate kiss in the start of your relationship that would have been the trigger for your desire. It's about bringing sexual currency, without any pressure for that to go anywhere, and trying to create a culture of high sexual currency.

What parts of life, or even love, can squash desire? We know from large scale data, like The British National Survey of Sexual Attitudes and Lifestyles research, that as a society we're having less sex now than we were having three decades ago. **Although frequency of sex is not a marker of a good sex life, it does tell us something about our busy lives.** I think we're getting really used to constant stimulation. And we're struggling more and more to just be together in a space where we're connected—not in a space where we're all on our devices. If we can't sit with our body and feel what's happening in our body, we're also missing a lot of organic cues for desire. The physical arousal for people of all genders is peaking and troughing throughout the day. Sometimes it's easier for penis owners to be more aware of it because they have more of a visible cue. But actually it happens for all people, with all bodies, that we get this peaking and troughing of arousal over the day or over the month—it sometimes connects to the menstrual cycle as well.

And just general tiredness, monotony, and the fullness of life are all factors. A lot of people are quite exhausted and come home after a long workday and then have lots of tasks to do, and then have work on their mind, so expecting to feel like sex at bedtime is incredibly difficult. ∎

UNWELCOME THOUGHTS: DO NOT DISTURB

Body image concerns, the shopping list, and all types of things can pop into our heads, which are not conducive to sexy times. Developing ways of refocusing to the present can start with bringing your mind back to what you see, smell, hear, and feel—it's a technique that can be practiced from day to day and that brings you back to your body and your partner.

Another idea is to consciously decide to make the bedroom a place where you leave your concerns at the door. Make this space a place where your mind can relax: phones left outside, cozy lights instead of harsh lights.

Take goals off the table before the start. Pressure and a sole focus on orgasm can make it harder to achieve and can induce performance anxiety. Enjoy the moment rather than rushing towards orgasms. Masturbation has proven health benefits, releasing endorphins and relieving stress—and it can even be a natural painkiller to help with period cramps!

EFFORT

Recognizing that good sex doesn't always have to be a spontaneous moment of passion can be a relief. Good sex can just as much be something that's planned. For people with busy schedules, this can help to carve out some time together. For couples experiencing an unwanted dry spell, a mutual commitment to reignite the spark can be the first step towards connecting sexually again. For those who feel more comfortable with time to prepare, this gives them some comfort from the fact that they know they can get in the mindset for sex.

A CELEBRATION OF THE UNDERRATED KISS

BITING CHEEKY KISS

TOOTH CLASHING
HEAD BASHING
GLASSES CRASHING KISS

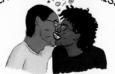

BACK OF THE HAND KISS

EROTIC NECK KISS

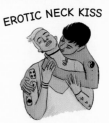

CARING
FOREHEAD KISS

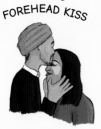

AFFECTIONATE SHOULDER
KISS

DELICATE
SOFT KISS

WELCOME KISS

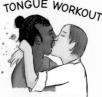

TONGUE WORKOUT

DEMENTOR'S KISS

GOODBYE, THANK YOU
FOR EVERYTHING
KISS

PLANT A KISS
(ON A PLANT)

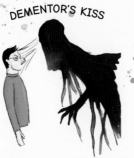

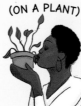

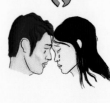

KISS WITH
ALL THE CHEMISTRY

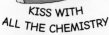

PECK ON THE LIPS

KISS FROM HEAD TO TOE

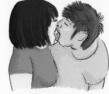

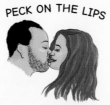

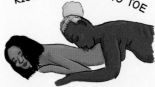

TIPSY KISS

WHY DON'T I WANT SEX?

Our desire for sex is dependent on many factors. It's okay not to be wanting sex all the time, or even at all. But if you're having a dry spell and are feeling like it is a problem, here are some questions to consider . . .

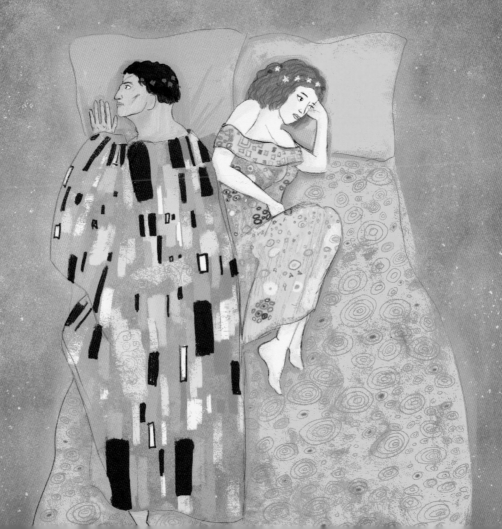

ARE YOU FEELING SOCIAL PRESSURE TO HAVE MORE SEX?

It feels like we're constantly being told that everyone else is having more sex than we are, and we should be having a certain amount of sex, otherwise something is wrong. But what *actually* feels right for you (and your partner/s)? When it comes to sex, as with most things, quality trumps quantity.

In the previous chapter, I interviewed the author Karen Gurney, also known as the Sex Doctor (see page 56), and according to her:

> "Most people assume they should be having sex about three times a week. And that statistic—no one knows where that's come from. But I can tell you that everyone says it. Everyone thinks they should be having sex a lot more than they do, but a third of people have had no sex at all in the last month. I think people become obsessed with frequency because it's something that people can mark their sex life against and say, 'I have an okay sex life.' **Every time you have sex that's not rewarding for one or both of you [in a relationship], it's chipping away at your desire, because sex has to be rewarding for us to want to do it.'**

ARE YOU EXPERIENCING THE KIND OF SEX YOU WANT?

Perhaps you're having the kind of sex that you think you should be having, or think your partner wants, but are not asking yourself what *you* want. "Good sex" is something to experience rather than perform. If you learn that sex isn't a place where your pleasure is given importance, then it's natural that you won't want it.

It could be a communication issue. We expect people to know what we want, but often there's a disconnect or a lack of communication, as it's hard to talk about it. Sometimes it's easier to perform than to confront and discuss your desires in sex. Unfortunately, mind-reading isn't a skill that we've evolved yet. A little friendly guidance can go a long way.

Maybe you're on different pages— you're just not into the same things. Everyone has different preferences and that's natural.

Perhaps your sexual partner just doesn't care about your pleasure. That's a hard truth, but if you've tried communicating, and sex still feels very one-sided and unpleasurable for you, then maybe the other person really doesn't care.

OTHERS AREN'T DOING IT AS MUCH AS YOU THINK

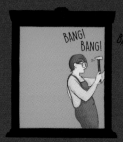
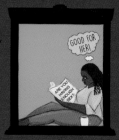
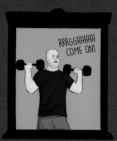
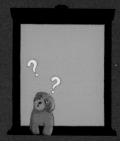
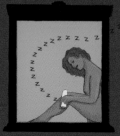
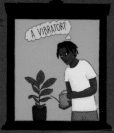
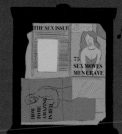
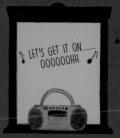
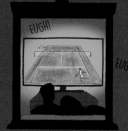
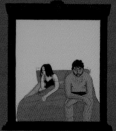
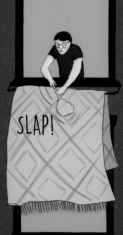
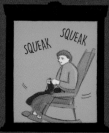
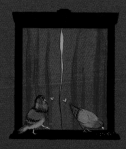
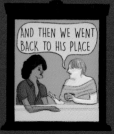
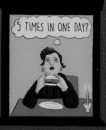

IS SOMETHING ELSE GOING ON IN OTHER ASPECTS OF YOUR LIFE?

Libido is affected by stress, and it's normal for it to disappear when you're experiencing stress. Perhaps your brain is busy, focusing on so many other things, so sex is the last thing on your mind. Some mental health problems like depression can also affect libido. Menopause and perimenopause, too! Anything that's playing with your sex hormones—such as medication or contraception—can also increase/decrease your desire for sex. It can be a tricky balance.

Not feeling good in your body can also affect the desire to have sex. When you feel unattractive, or are concerned with how you look during sex, it can keep your head in a state of worrying about what the other person is thinking.

IS LACK OF SEX A PROBLEM FOR YOU?

If you're in a sexless relationship and it is a problem for one of you, then something should change. Look at how to reconnect or discuss the possibility of seeing a sex therapist to provide further advice. But if you're both okay with not having the same sexual connection, then that's all right. If the relationship is working for you, then it's no one else's business! Some people are in asexual partnerships and don't desire sex. If you're questioning whether you may be on the asexual spectrum, there is an interview on page 87 which gives a more in-depth look at asexuality.

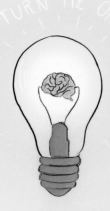

THE BRAIN IS THE LARGEST
SEXUAL ORGAN IN THE BODY

SHOULD SEX HURT?

The first time often hurts because of nerves, lack of lubrication, and lack of effort/understanding of female arousal, but the belief that it *should* hurt is harmful and normalizes pain.

It's not uncommon for sex to hurt the first few times, but if it continues to be painful, this may be for a number of reasons. Please know that there is help out there, and communities that can be affirming and let you know you are not alone. Sex educator Debby Herbenick conducted a study which showed that 30 percent of women report pain during vaginal sex, and 72 percent during anal sex.

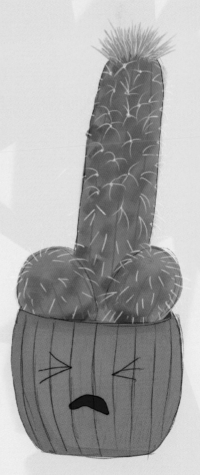

FIRST UP: LUBE!

USING LUBE IS NOT SHAMEFUL!

Friction can be a cause of pain and discomfort during sex, and lube is here just for that, to provide extra slip for all types of sex— solo, vaginal, anal—and some even double as a massage oil.

WATER BASED

✓ Good for use with toys

✓ Safe to use with condoms

✗ Can be a bit sticky

OIL BASED

✓ Long lasting

✗ Not for use with latex condoms as can increase risk of tears

✗ Associated with higher rates of candida (which could lead to yeast infection)

SILICONE BASED

✓ Long lasting

✓ Safe for use with condoms

✓ Anal sex

✗ Can degrade silicone toys

HYBRID

✓ Mix of water-based and silicone/oil

✓ Long lasting

✓ Easy to clean off, reactivates with water (not spit)

LOOK FOR PH-BALANCED LUBES

Check ingredients

Flavoring and scents are more likely to contain irritants that can upset the vaginal biome!

EDIBLE LUBES

Edible lube can be swallowed in small quantities

Flavored doesn't necessarily mean edible

CHECK EXPIRATION DATE!

NATURAL ≠ SAFE

GENITAL ISSUES

LET'S TALK VAGINISMUS

Vaginismus is a psychosexual condition where penetration is incredibly painful or even impossible, due to an involuntary contraction of the vaginal muscles/pelvic floor. Tampons, smear-test speculums, fingers, and penises can be difficult, or impossible, to insert. Primary vaginismus is where penetration has never been possible; this is often discovered when first trying to insert a tampon or have penetrative sex. No one's story is the same, but often narratives are linked to shame or fear around sex—no wonder, when women and people with vulvas are discouraged from exploring their sexuality and are told the first time should hurt and draw blood. Secondary vaginismus is when penetration has happened before, but due to a situation or change—perhaps trauma, surgery, gynecological cancers, menopause, or something else— vaginismus develops.

The sensation of penetration for those with vaginismus has been compared to being cut with a knife, and even to it feeling like there's a brick wall allowing nothing in. It's a vicious cycle, because once pain has been experienced, the mind will feel less safe and the vaginal muscles will be less likely to be able to relax.

Vaginismus is widely misunderstood, even by some medical professionals, and the advice that people with the condition often hear is to "just relax," which can make them feel even more isolated and like they're the only person experiencing it. However, as it is said to affect two in 1,000 people (and even that figure is probably under-representative), vaginismus is much more common than you think.

Luckily, there are a few options to look into for treatment, so all hope is not lost if you want to overcome it:

· **Using dilators** (a set of vaginal trainers, which come in a range of sizes) to get the vagina used to having things inserted (nothing to do with stretching). *Tip: use them with a vibrator to make the experience feel pleasurable rather than medical.*

· **Sex therapy (talking)** to help you understand and change your feelings about your body and sex.

· **Pelvic floor therapy**, including breathing exercises and pelvic floor massage.

VULVODYNIA AND VULVAL PAIN

Vulvodynia is characterized by a long-lasting burning and itching pain on the vulva, which doesn't have a clear cause. It can be excruciating, causing pain, not only during sex but at other times, too. The pain may be there all the time or may come and go. There's a lot of crossover with vaginismus, and people may have both. Many doctors will say there's no cure, but there are a few options to look into that may help to manage the symptoms: eating a diet rich in probiotics, applying cool ice packs, wearing cotton underwear, or using lidocaine, a local anesthetic agent.

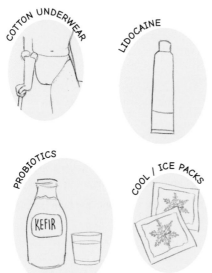

ENDOMETRIOSIS

This occurs when tissue similar to the lining of the womb grows in other places. It can cause many symptoms, including pain during and after sex, as well as excruciating periods.

OVARIAN CYSTS

These are fluid-filled sacs that grow on the ovaries. Most are harmless and disappear in a few months, although some cysts can grow large, cause a lot of pain and discomfort, and need to be surgically removed.

FIBROIDS

Non-cancerous growths that develop in the womb may cause symptoms in one in three people, such as heavy painful periods, lower back pain, a need to urinate more, and pain during sex.

VAGINAL DRYNESS

The most common cause is a drop in estrogen, from menopause, breastfeeding, or childbirth, although other factors such as medication could cause dryness as well.

LICHEN SCLEROSUS

When the genital skin becomes scaly and inflamed, with itchy white patches; prescription steroid creams can help relieve the symptoms.

PAINFUL BLADDER SYNDROME

This is difficult to diagnose, but symptoms include intense pelvic pain, the need to pee more than usual, and pain when the bladder is filling up.

PELVIC FLOOR DYSFUNCTION

An inability to correctly relax and control your pelvic floor muscles to have a bowel movement. It can result in incontinence, constipation, and straining to defecate.

PELVIC ADHESION

Scar tissue that can cause organs to become stuck together.

PREVIOUS INJURIES

Such as vaginal tears from giving birth.

VAGINITIS

Vaginal inflammation, especially yeast or bacterial overgrowth in the vagina, can cause itching and irritation.

PHIMOSIS

When the foreskin is tight and gets stuck over the head of the penis and can't be pulled fully back. It is normal in babies and toddlers; for adults, it can cause painful erections and urinary tract infections (UTIs). It may occur for a number of reasons, including poor hygiene, skin conditions such as eczema, injuries, or infections. If it's not manageable, steroid creams can be prescribed to loosen the skin or, in severe cases, part-circumcisions may be recommended.

PARAPHIMOSIS

Where the foreskin gets stuck behind the head of the penis and can cut off the circulation. This is an emergency, whereas phimosis isn't. To reduce the risks, wash and dry the head and foreskin regularly and put the foreskin back into its resting place.

A NOTE ABOUT ANAL SEX

Anal sex should be done with preparation and lube, and often with more discussion than for other types of sex.

The muscles need to relax, which lube and massage can help with.

Prepare for a bit of poop. You can wash beforehand with water and soap, but enemas can be dangerous—irritating the cells in the rectum, generating excess mucus, and causing dryness.

It should be enjoyable for both people.

You can get pregnant from anal sex—if the clean-up afterwards isn't done carefully, the semen can drip and get inside the vagina.

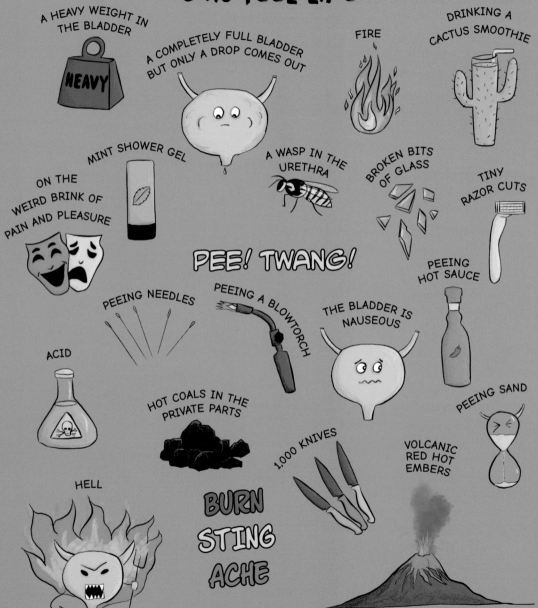

IRRITATION, INFECTIONS, STIs, AND UTIs

There is a whole host of reasons why sex could hurt! Our genitals are complicated things. The natural biomes can be easily irritated by feminine washes, tight underwear, vaginal douching, and spermicides, and latex condoms can give some people an allergy—so avoid feminine washes, get cotton underwear, and use latex-free condoms if you're experiencing problems.

Sexually transmitted infections (STIs) can also cause pain and itching, so if a new pain has developed, it can be handy to get an STI check to rule them out.

Pain after sex can take the form of a UTI (urinary tract infection), whereby a build-up of bacteria gets into the urethra. **Tips to reduce the risk are to pee after sex, wipe from front to back after going to the toilet, and drink plenty of fluids.** Some people are more prone to getting these infections and may suffer from chronic UTIs and need antibiotics to help manage them.

Let's focus on having enjoyable, pain free sex! Painful sex is a sign that something isn't right. Don't push through pain for someone else—take penetrative sex off the menu. And when something does feel painful or not right, check in with your doctor or healthcare professional. You can also try to understand your own symptoms and see whether there's anything online that resonates with you.

THINGS THAT IRRITATE THE VAGINAL MICROBIOME

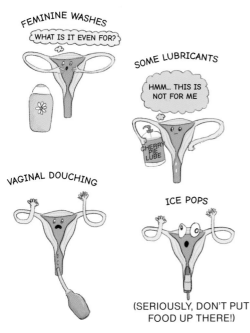

FEMININE WASHES

WHAT IS IT EVEN FOR?

SOME LUBRICANTS

HMM... THIS IS NOT FOR ME

CHERRY PIE LUBE

VAGINAL DOUCHING

ICE POPS

(SERIOUSLY, DON'T PUT FOOD UP THERE!)

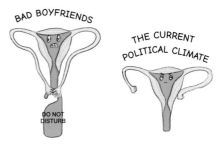

BAD BOYFRIENDS

DO NOT DISTURB

THE CURRENT POLITICAL CLIMATE

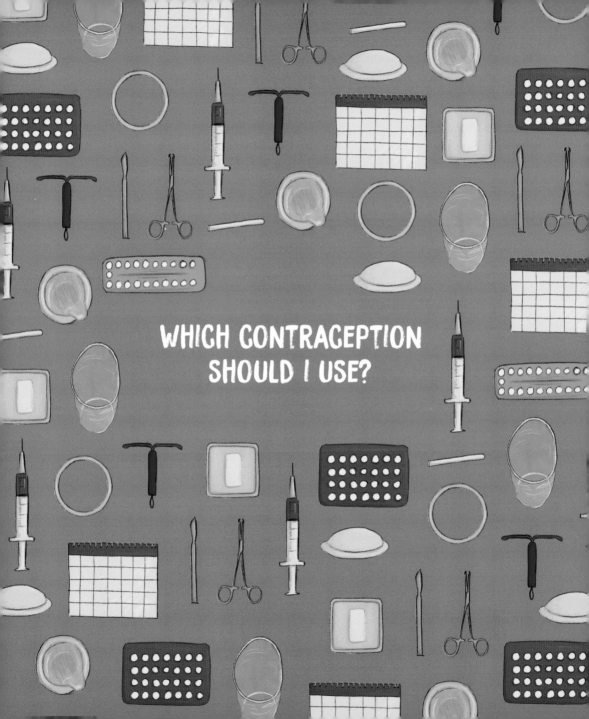

WHICH CONTRACEPTION
SHOULD I USE?

Contraception can be a big part of a sexually active person's life. When protecting yourself from STIs or wanting to avoid getting pregnant, contraception is key, yet there's a lack of awareness about how many options are out there. I hear so many stories of people on contraception that made them feel depressed or lose their sex drive completely, and of others who reacted awfully to one form, but found that another was life-changing!

Here are the options, and some pros and cons to consider to help you decide what is right for you. Ultimately, everyone's circumstances are different, and medical professionals can offer essential insights based on access to your medical records.

SOME THINGS YOU MAY WANT TO CONSIDER—IF YOU WANT PERIODS, HOW OFTEN YOU WANT TO THINK ABOUT CONTRACEPTION, EFFECTIVENESS, AND THE PROS + THE CONS.

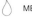 MENSTRUATION   FREQUENCY   TYPICAL EFFECTIVENESS AT PROS + CONS
PREVENTING PREGNANCY

HORMONAL METHODS

COMBINED PILL

A small pill that contains estrogen and progesterone. It works by preventing the ovaries from releasing an egg each month, thickening cervical mucus (making it harder for sperm to swim), and by thinning the lining of the womb, so there's much less chance of a fertilized egg settling and growing.

 Period may be lighter and the combined pill could ease period pain

 Taken at the same time every day, with a week off to allow for your period

 91 percent

 Period may become lighter and less painful. Requires daily remembering. You can decide whether you take the week off for your period. It is not suitable for everyone, due to a small risk of blood clots, so a general checkup is recommended before starting. Potential side effects include lower sex drive, changes in mood, and breast soreness. Linked to increased risk of breast cancer, and decreased risk of ovarian, uterine, and colon cancer. No protection against STIs.

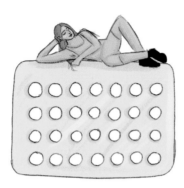

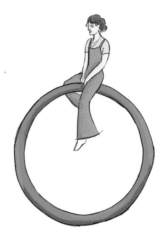

MINI PILL

A small pill containing only progestin. This works by thickening cervical mucus, making it harder for sperm to swim, and by thinning the lining of the womb, so there's much less chance of a fertilized egg settling and growing.

- Some progestin-only pills also stop your ovaries producing eggs while you're taking it, and may reduce or stop your periods altogether

- Taken at the same time every day, without breaks

- 92 percent

- An option if you want to take the pill but can't take estrogen. Requires daily remembering. Rare but potential side effects include acne, increased or decreased sex drive, changes in mood, breast soreness, and cysts on ovaries. No protection against STIs.

THE RING

A hormonal contraceptive providing estrogen and progestin through a ring placed in the vagina. It works by preventing the ovaries from releasing an egg each month, thickening cervical mucus, making it harder for sperm to swim, and by thinning the lining of the womb, so there's much less chance of a fertilized egg settling and growing.

- Periods may become lighter and less painful

- Changed every three weeks, with a week ring-free to allow for your period

- 91 percent

- Don't have to think about it daily. Potential side effects include spotting, breast soreness, changes in mood and sex drive, and a small chance of blood clots. Small increased risk of breast cancer and cervical cancer. No protection against STIs.

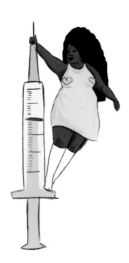

INJECTABLE

A hormonal form of contraception (progestin), this works by stopping the ovaries from releasing an egg, thickening cervical fluid so that sperm can't get through as easily, and thinning the uterine lining, which makes it harder for a fertilized egg to settle and grow.

 Can make periods irregular, lighter, heavier, or shorter, and for some people periods stop altogether

 Every three months, from your healthcare provider

 97 percent

 An option if you can't take estrogen. Don't have to think about it daily. Periods may become irregular. Potential side effects include acne, hair loss, and changes in mood and sex drive, and it may take months to wear off, so is not ideal for those who know they may want to get pregnant soon. Small risk of infection at the site of injection. No protection against STIs.

CONTRACEPTIVE PATCH

A hormonal contraceptive, providing estrogen and progestin through the skin with a sticker that can be placed on the butt, upper body, or lower abdomen. It works by preventing the ovaries from releasing an egg each month, thickening cervical mucus (making it harder for sperm to swim), and by thinning the lining of the womb, so there's much less chance of a fertilized egg settling and growing.

 Periods may be lighter and less painful

 Applied once a week for three weeks, with a week off to allow you to have your period

 92 percent

 Period may become lighter and less painful. Potential side effects include spotting, breast tenderness, changes in mood and sex drive, and a small chance of blood clots. Can cause skin irritation. No protection against STIs.

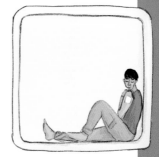

LONG–ACTING REVERSIBLE METHODS

HORMONAL IUD

A healthcare provider inserts the T-shaped intrauterine device (IUD) into the uterus. It releases the hormone progestin, which thickens the cervical mucus so that sperm can't get through as easily, thins the lining of the womb, and for some people can prevent eggs from being produced in the ovaries.

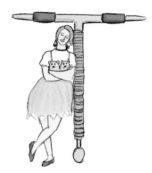

 Periods may become heavier and more painful in the first three to six months

 Can last for up to five years

 99 percent

 An option if you can't take estrogen. Don't have to think about it often at all. This method also gives a low level of hormone. Insertion of the IUD can be painful, and there may be irregular bleeding and sometimes mood changes. In rare cases there are ectopic pregnancies, or the IUD could go through the wall of the uterus during insertion. No protection against STIs.

COPPER IUD

A healthcare provider inserts the T-shaped intrauterine device (IUD) into the uterus. Unlike the hormonal IUD, this is hormone-free; instead, the copper prevents both egg and sperm from surviving in the womb.

 Periods may become heavier and more painful in the first three to six months

 Can last for up to ten years

 99 percent

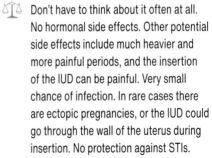 Don't have to think about it often at all. No hormonal side effects. Other potential side effects include much heavier and more painful periods, and the insertion of the IUD can be painful. Very small chance of infection. In rare cases there are ectopic pregnancies, or the IUD could go through the wall of the uterus during insertion. No protection against STIs.

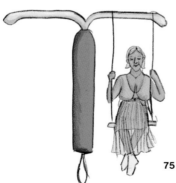

IMPLANT

A small bit of plastic that is inserted just under the skin of your arm. It contains the hormone progestin, which thickens the cervical mucus so that sperm can't get through as easily, and thins the lining of the womb.

 Can help make periods lighter and less painful, or they may be irregular or stop all together

 Can last for up to three years

 99 percent

 An option if you can't take estrogen. Don't have to think about it often at all. It can help make periods lighter and less painful. Potential side effects include irregular bleeding, acne, plus changes in mood and sex drive. No protection against STIs.

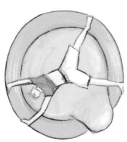

BARRIER METHODS

CONDOM

A sheath that covers the penis or lines the vagina, collects sperm, and prevents it from entering the vagina. It can also prevent the transmission of most STIs if used correctly during vaginal, anal, or oral sex.

 Not applicable

 Single use and should be disposed of afterwards

 85 percent

 They are widely available and often free at your doctor's office. They can prevent both pregnancy and STIs. They are hormone free, don't alter your fertility, and don't have physical side effects. Possible disadvantages include a possible reduction in sensitivity during intercourse. Tearing/damage could occur to the condom, making them ineffective, and they can expire.

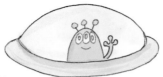

DIAPHRAGM

A shallow cup that is inserted into the vagina (up to three hours before sex) to cover the cervix and is used with a spermicide (cream that kills sperm).

◌ Not applicable

◷ Must be left in for six hours after having sex for the spermicide to work. There are different sizes, and they need to be cleaned after use and checked for holes before using them again.

⟳ 84 percent

⚖ Diaphragms are hormone free, and offer skin-on-skin contact and some protection against STIs. Possible disadvantages are that spermicides may cause allergic reactions, and it can take time to master the technique of putting the diaphragm in.

DENTAL DAM

A latex or polyurethane sheet, used for contact between mouth and vagina/anus to protect against exchanging fluids and some STIs.

◌ Not applicable

◷ Single-use

⟳ Not applicable

⚖ Dental dams are hormone free and offer some protection against STIs. Unfortunately they can be harder to source than condoms.

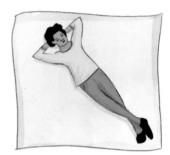

PRE-EXPOSURE PROPHYLAXIS (PrEP)

This is not technically contraception, but is a way to prevent contracting HIV by taking a daily antiretroviral pill (a class of drug that stops the activity of retroviruses). If a person is exposed to HIV, the PrEP drugs will prevent HIV entering the cells. You can stop and start PrEP safely, but it takes seven to twenty-two days of daily use for full effectiveness to resume. This can be a good option for a person who is having sex with someone with HIV or others who are at a high risk of contracting HIV.

OTHER METHODS

STERILIZATION

Female sterilization works by applying clamp-like clips or restrictive silicone rings over the fallopian tubes, or by tying, cutting, and removing a small piece of the fallopian tube. Male sterilization works by cutting, blocking, or sealing the tubes that carry sperm from the testicles to the semen, so that the semen will contain no sperm.

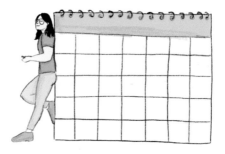

 Not applicable

 Permanent

 Over 99 percent

Both procedures are very difficult to reverse, and it is not always possible to do so, so be really sure you don't want children/any more children. With female sterilization, there is a very small risk of complications including infection and organ damage, and occasionally fallopian tubes can rejoin. With male sterilization there is a small risk of complications including blood inside the scrotum, hard lumps, and infection, and in very rare circumstances the vas deferens tubes can reconnect. No protection against STIs.

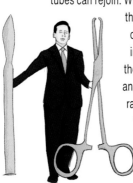

NATURAL FAMILY PLANNING

Fertility tracking is where female temperature, discharge, and the menstrual cycle are all monitored to predict when ovulation is occurring.

 Not applicable

 Requires daily monitoring

 76 percent

 It can take a few months to understand your body's patterns, and stress and illness can interrupt cycles and make ovulation much harder to predict. It works for people who are open to having a baby—and, crucially, for anyone who is okay with exposure to STIs (or who is in a monogamous relationship in which both/all partners have been tested for STIs). It requires a lot of self-control and body awareness. Note: pre-ejaculate can contain sperm.

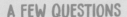

WHEN SHOULD I GET STI CHECKS?

STIs are passed through unprotected sexual contact; some of them have signs and symptoms, but many don't, so it's important to get checked when having unprotected sex. It may be worth testing in between partners if you're able to, or at three-month intervals, to capture early symptom onset for key infections. You can get checked through urgent care clinics, your doctor, or even by ordering kits online. Checks may involve urine samples, blood tests, a swab of the urethra and/or vagina, and a look at your genitals.

CAN I GET PREGNANT FROM SEX WITHOUT PENETRATION?

This is possible, if ejaculation happens near your vagina or if there's been contact between an erect penis and the vagina. However, as sperm don't survive for long outside the body, the chances of pregnancy are very low.

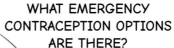

WHAT EMERGENCY CONTRACEPTION OPTIONS ARE THERE?

For unprotected sex or when your contraception method has failed, there is the emergency contraceptive pill (morning-after pill) and the IUD.

Getting an IUD up to 5 days after sex is the most effective method with 1 percent chance of pregnancy.

The morning-after pill prevents pregnancy for up to five days after having unprotected sex with 89 percent effectiveness, but it requires a prescription.

Brand names of morning-after pills include Plan B One Step, My Way, EContra, Take Action, AfterPill, Option 2, Preventeza, My Choice, and Aftera. These levonorgestrel pills can lower your chance of getting pregnant by 75 to 89 percent if taken it within three days after unprotected sex.

CAN I GET PREGNANT ON MY PERIOD?

It is possible, but it's unlikely. Sperm can survive for up to seven days, so if ovulation happens early, pregnancy may occur.

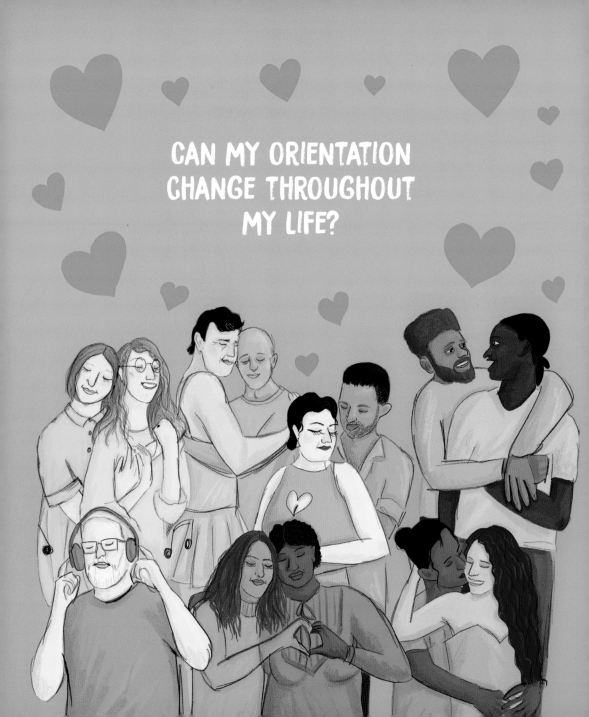

CAN MY ORIENTATION
CHANGE THROUGHOUT
MY LIFE?

SEXUAL FLUIDITY

There is an expectation that we will discover our orientation early on, and that it will be set in stone forever. While this is the case for many, that doesn't happen for everyone. The idea that your sexuality can change has historically been used against queer people, with some extreme manifestations of this mindset including the invention and practice of conversion therapy.

While our sexuality is not chosen, it can change throughout our lifetime, for some people due to external events or by just . . . changing. Your feelings now don't discount anything you felt before and what you felt before doesn't discount your feelings now.

UNPICKING HETERONORMATIVITY

If you're brought up in an environment that taught you that homosexuality—or, more generally, queerness—is wrong and sinful, then you might internalize, and learn these scripts, too. For most people, heteronormative ideals have been presented as the standard since childhood. This can be why people discover or come to terms with their sexuality later in life, after unpicking what they've learned.

SEXUAL AND ROMANTIC ORIENTATION EXISTS ON A SPECTRUM

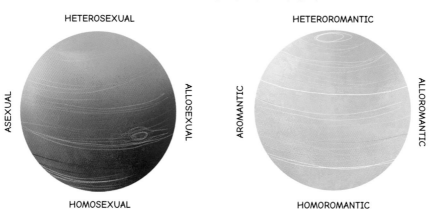

HETEROSEXUAL

ASEXUAL — ALLOSEXUAL

HOMOSEXUAL

HETEROROMANTIC

AROMANTIC — ALLOROMANTIC

HOMOROMANTIC

QUEER MYTHS

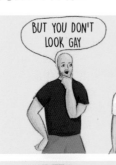
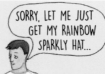
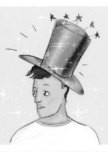

SOMEONE'S SEXUALITY DOESN'T HAVE TO FIT YOUR STEREOTYPE OF A CERTAIN LOOK

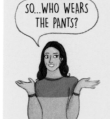
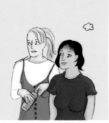
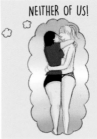

SOMEONE'S RELATIONSHIP DOESN'T HAVE TO FIT YOUR HETERONORMATIVE MODEL OF "MAN AND WOMAN"

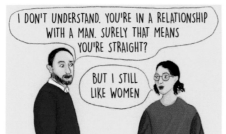
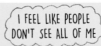
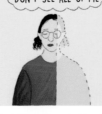

IDENTITY ISN'T DEPENDENT ON WHO YOU'RE DATING

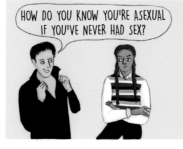
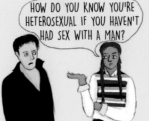

PEOPLE DON'T OWE YOU PROOF OF ORIENTATION

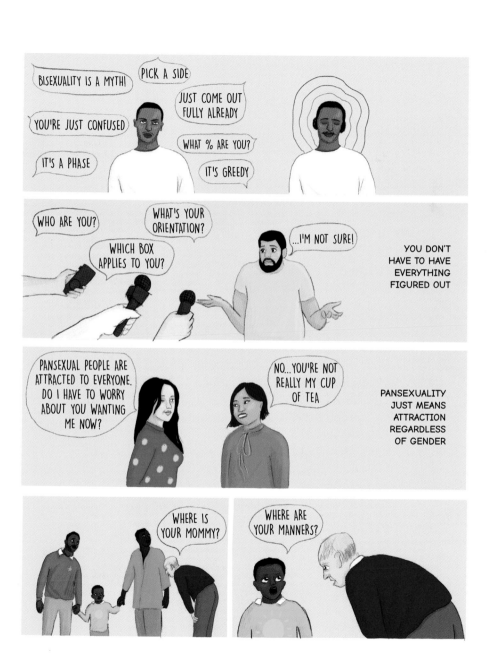

COMING OUT

You don't owe anyone your coming out. A conception of queerness that hinges on your coming out is very reductive. For some people, coming out is necessary, feels right, and provides liberation; for others, it's not right for them, may not feel needed, or might not be safe. You don't have to come out to be queer, and you can prioritize your wellbeing over a need to come out. You can reveal it to a few trusted people and not everyone. The ultimate symbol of queerness shouldn't be coming out, but for queer people to live their best lives, whatever that means *to them*.

If coming out is an important step for you, the charity Brook has some excellent advice . . .

1. **For some people it might be a step or an event, while for others it might be an ongoing process.**
2. **You don't have to come out to everyone all at once.** Consider who you think would be supportive. Maybe write a letter before speaking face to face.
3. **Connect with others** in community groups facing similar challenges, for extra support.
4. **If someone's initial reaction is negative**, it doesn't mean they'll feel that way forever; they may need some time to process it.
5. **Prioritize your own comfort, happiness, and safety**, and come out only if and when it feels right for you.

SEXUALITY AND ROMANCE TERMINOLOGY

Language is constantly evolving and changing, and there may be other terms that are welcomed in soon, so this list does not encompass the totality of language that may be used to express sexuality and attraction.

Alloromantic: someone who experiences romantic attraction

Allosexual: someone who experiences sexual attraction

Aromantic (aro): feeling little to no romantic attraction

Asexual (ace): feeling little to no sexual attraction

Biromantic (bi): often means having romantic feelings towards your gender and at least one other

Bisexual (bi): often means being sexually attracted to your gender and at least one other

Demiromantic (demi): feeling a lack of romantic attraction to others until there's an emotional connection built

Demisexual (demi): feeling a lack of sexual attraction until there's an emotional connection built

Fluid (sexually/romantically): not in a fixed state

Gay or homosexual: men who are sexually attracted to men, women who are sexually attracted to women

Gray-asexual: the gray area between asexuality and sexuality

Heteronormative: the view that heterosexuality is the preferred orientation

Heteroromantic: men romantically attracted to women, women romantically attracted to men

Heterosexual/straight: men sexually attracted to women, women sexually attracted to men

Lesbian: women exclusively attracted to women (this can also include non-binary people)

Non-labeled: someone who doesn't use a label to identify others

Omnisexual: being attracted to all genders, with gender playing a role in the attraction

Panromantic: often means having romantic feelings regardless of gender

Pansexual: often means having sexual feelings regardless of gender

Polysexual: attracted to multiple genders

Queer: a term reclaimed by the LGBTQIA+ community as an umbrella term to cover the range of orientations and habits of the non-exclusively heterosexual majority.

Questioning: someone who is unsure of their sexual orientation (or gender identity)

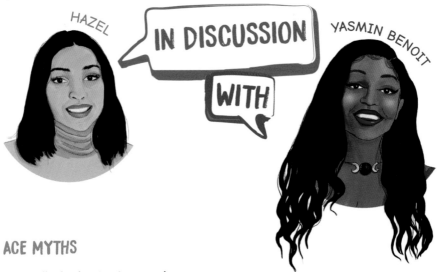

ACE MYTHS

Asexuality is about not, or rarely, experiencing sexual attraction. You can still be attracted to people in other ways: romantically, intellectually, aesthetically. There are quite a few myths about asexuality, so I asked the British asexual campaigner, writer, and model Yasmin Benoit about some of these.

Why do you think asexuality is still so invisible and taboo? It's a combination of things. Our conversations about sexuality have diversified a lot recently. But they've diversified and progressed in that way because it's been necessary for their legislative protection because [those with certain orientations] were systematically oppressed.

And consequently, in the battle for those changes, we've had to talk about those specific orientations more, and lots of those conversations have been driven by mainstream, widely accepted discrimination, which is not something that the ace community has had to deal with on the same level. So consequently we haven't had as much of a reason to push, and people haven't had as much of a reason to pay attention.

Also, we kind of went from a very sort of conservative mindset towards sexuality, and now we've swung in a much more liberal, sex-positive direction. And based on the way we've been taught to conceptualize sex positivity and liberation, it doesn't really align with people who are associated with not having sex. So it's seen as not really being part of the conversation, because people are interpreting asexuality as just a bunch of people who don't have sex and have nothing really to contribute. The act of not experiencing sexuality in that way is seen as being a sign of a less liberated way to live. It doesn't tend to kind of fit with the way the movement is presented.

What do you think are the most common misconceptions and myths surrounding asexuality?

I feel like they're all based around there being something physically or mentally wrong with you: that it's some kind of physical disorder, or the kind of thing that can be solved with medication; or it's hormone-related or biological; or it's something pathological, like a mental illness, or a side effect of a mental illness. Or that it's a personality trait or the consequence of trauma or a bad experience. Or that it's a reflection of your personal views; that you are a prude or anti-sex, or you're "unliberated," and that's why your sexuality has turned out like that.

Have you experienced any microaggressions? And do you have any responses that others can use?

There's so many—it's been twenty years; the regurgitation of old homophobic rhetoric:
- "You just haven't found the right person yet."

- "You're too young to know what your orientation is."
- "Someone will unlock that part of your sexuality one day."
- "You don't look asexual."

The common one I hear is, "You can't know you're asexual unless you've actually had sex." To that—especially if a straight guy says that—I'm like, "In that case, you don't know you're straight unless you've had gay sex, because you've got to apply that logic to everyone."

Do you have any advice for someone who might be questioning whether they're asexual?

It can be hard to understand what sexual attraction is if you haven't experienced it. I often hear asexual people who are questioning their identity saying things like, "Was this sexual attraction?", but it's hard to recognize if it's something you don't feel or really understand. The question is: do you want to involve someone in your sexuality based on your own natural inclination rather than because you feel like you're meant to? And if the answer is no, then that's kind of an ace thing. In the grand scheme of things, it's not a big deal. You can still live a perfectly happy, fulfilling life. The terminology is useful. Use it, if you find it helpful. If you don't, there's no obligation. Just make your peace with it and then live your life. ∎

HOW DOES CONSENT WORK?

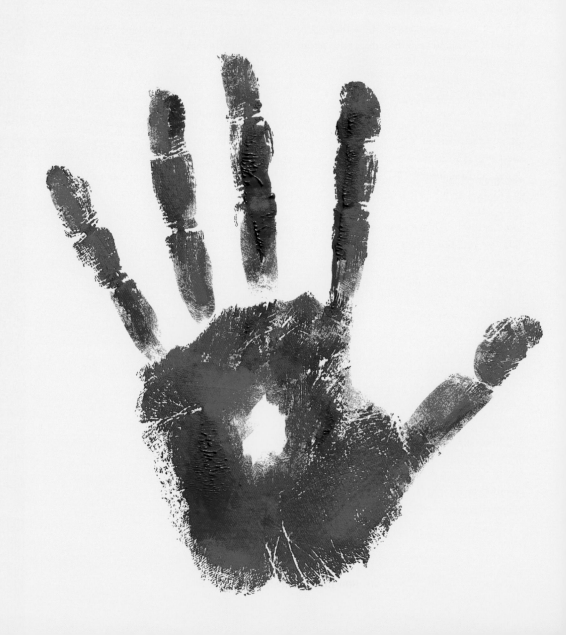

According to U.S. Code 920, Article 120, "The term 'consent' means a freely given agreement to the conduct at issue by a competent person. An expression of lack of consent through words or conduct means there is no consent. Lack of verbal or physical resistance does not constitute consent." But, as conveyed by Michaela Coel in her hit TV show on sexual dynamics *I May Destroy You*, the reality is more complex.

ENTHUSIASTIC CONSENT

Consent is often oversimplified to statements such as "Just say no" and "Be clear and assertive," as if it's always that easy. This rhetoric in itself is an example of victim blaming—like if you went along with something, or put up with something, it's your fault. Someone may say yes, but if they are in a situation of fear, don't feel safe to say no, or are being forced or manipulated, then they don't have the freedom to make that choice. Someone may consent to one thing, but not to something else. It's almost like people have tried fixing sexual assault by providing a formula for how not to be assaulted. In reality, consent can be withdrawn at any time.

Enthusiastic consent focuses on excitement towards a proposition, rather than uncertainty. People communicate through both body language and words, so both matter.

"We live in a world where sperm banks have a right to reject sperm but wombs don't. Where driving while drunk is a crime, but raping while drunk is an excuse. Where trespassing private property is a red line, but violating a woman's body is a gray area. We live in a world that chooses what and who to protect; where we're told it's not that simple, but it is.'"

FARIDA D., AUTHOR OF *THE 10TH LIST OF SHIT THAT MADE ME A FEMINIST*

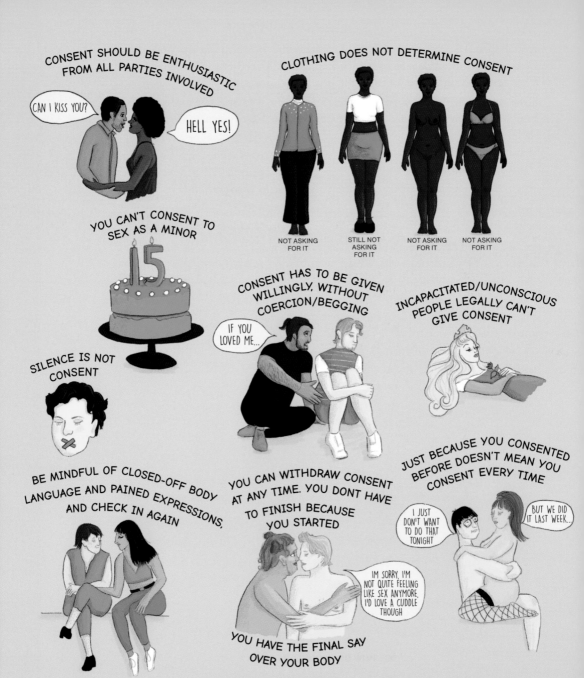

BDSM* *(BONDAGE, DISCIPLINE/DOMINATION, SADISM/SUBMISSION, MASOCHISM)

While there are plenty of bad examples of BDSM online, BDSM culture actually has consent at its core—it has to! The BDSM community often turns to contracts and communication ahead of an act to understand desires, and uses safe words throughout to check in, as well as being aware of the power dynamics that also affect the relationship. Perhaps even those who don't have an interest in those practices could, through this, find guidance on how to seek confirmation of consent in a way that maintains the sexiness and spontaneity.

There are some people who just don't know all the nuances around consent because there was never any education. And many people don't really practice consent well in day-to-day life, either— think "Come on, just have one drink," or "Go on, give Auntie a hug," even after you said you didn't want to.

Certain people find reading body language difficult—for example, some people on the autistic spectrum may struggle with this. However, the law is binary: it's either consent or it's not, so where there is uncertainty it can be safer to check in with direct verbal questions such as "How much do you want to do this?" And if the response is "100 percent!" then you're good to go.

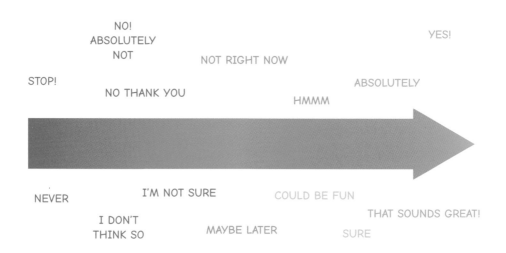

NO!
ABSOLUTELY
NOT

NOT RIGHT NOW

YES!

STOP!

NO THANK YOU

ABSOLUTELY

HMMM

NEVER

I'M NOT SURE

COULD BE FUN

THAT SOUNDS GREAT!

I DON'T
THINK SO

MAYBE LATER

SURE

A DARKER SIDE

A darker issue lies in the fact that some people don't truly care for consent; in fact, some people find a lack of consent sexy, or a challenge. It can be seen in the nature of those thinking that "no" means "convince me," and that women are always playing hard to get.

A recent example of this is the advent of revenge porn. A lot of those who purposely leak nudes derive pleasure from the fact that they are inherently non-consensual. Consent covers more than just the act itself: it is also necessary before sending a nude photo or filming someone.

A leaked video can end careers, cause bullying at school and slut-shaming, and have a lifelong impact. Yet often there are no consequences for the perpetrator. And when there are consequences, hate is often directed back at the victim. Imagine something very private being taken out of your control. However, as the scope of sex has expanded, the law is now increasingly on the cyber-victim's side. As of 2022, Congress allows victims of revenge porn to file civil claims in federal court against their perpetrators. Several states have also made "upskirting" (secretly taking photos or recording up someone's dress or skirt) illegal as well, hopefully with more to come.

TO REPORT OR NOT TO REPORT

In far too many cases of sexual assault and rape, survivors are treated like the criminals. There are more than 400,000 estimated rapes in the United States every year, with about a quarter of those reported to law enforcement. Only 0.7 percent resulted in a felony conviction for the perpetrator. With convictions so low, it's understandable that not everyone wants to come forward.

There seems to be a very small window to be classified as the "perfect victim." We see rape survivors scrutinized and dissected by the media. We hear of defense attorneys using past sexual history, the type of clothing worn, and explicit text messages to humiliate, gaslight, and undermine survivors, using insignificant facts to get away from the crime, to try to prove they were willing. This goes against the retractable nature of consent—you can be sex-positive, enjoy sex, and *still* not consent.

And when someone doesn't want to report an assault, it's completely understandable, no matter how unjust it may feel.

NO ONE DESERVES TO BE ASSAULTED OR RAPED— THE END

If you have experienced some form of sexual assault or rape, RAINN (Rape, Abuse & Incest National Network) offers resources, advice, and a free, anonymous helpline.

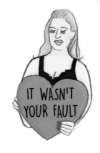

IT WASN'T YOUR FAULT

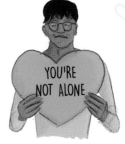

YOU'RE NOT ALONE

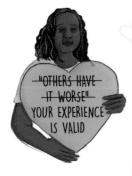

~~"OTHERS HAVE IT WORSE"~~ YOUR EXPERIENCE IS VALID

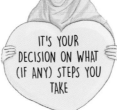

IT'S YOUR DECISION ON WHAT (IF ANY) STEPS YOU TAKE

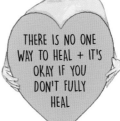

THERE IS NO ONE WAY TO HEAL + IT'S OKAY IF YOU DON'T FULLY HEAL

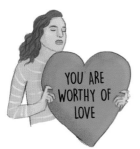

YOU ARE WORTHY OF LOVE

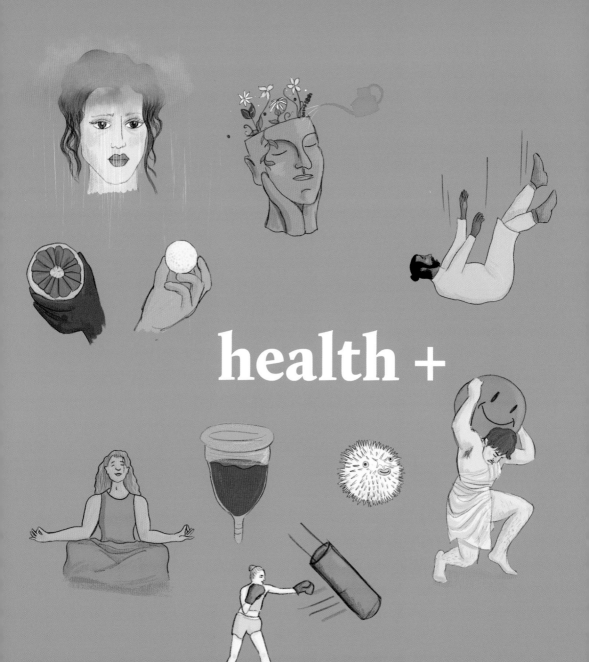

health +

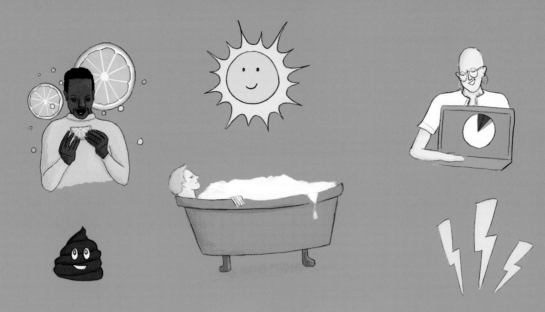

wellbeing

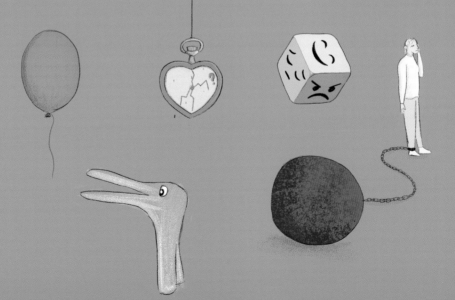

The pandemic was a global reminder of the fragility of our health and lives. We went through collective loss and grief, and were forced to face the impact of our mental and physical health, which made many of us re-evaluate what's important and how we are living our lives.

This section includes those niggling health questions that you might have and may turn to Google for. It also explores some of those deep, difficult topics that are part of the human experience, such as grief; digs into practical matters such as communicating with doctors; and takes a look at common wellbeing practices, such as reducing stress.

In this section I discuss the different types of common mental health issues, as well as some of the triggers for them. This includes interviews with three experts, bestselling author and psychotherapist Julia Samuel, who specializes in grief counseling, Anxiety Josh, bestselling author and therapist, and journalist and founder of The Femedic, Monica Karpinski.

This section of the book is packed with statistics and clinical advice on navigating mental health problems, which are by no means a substitute for full medical attention. However, I hope these words will help you feel seen, understood, or at least entertained for a moment.

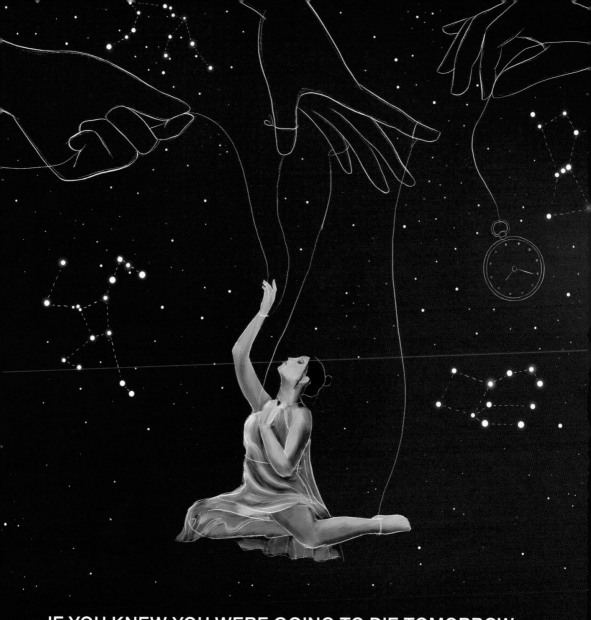

IF YOU KNEW YOU WERE GOING TO DIE TOMORROW
WHAT WOULD YOU DO TODAY?

DOES EVERYONE EXPERIENCE POOR MENTAL HEALTH AT SOME POINT?

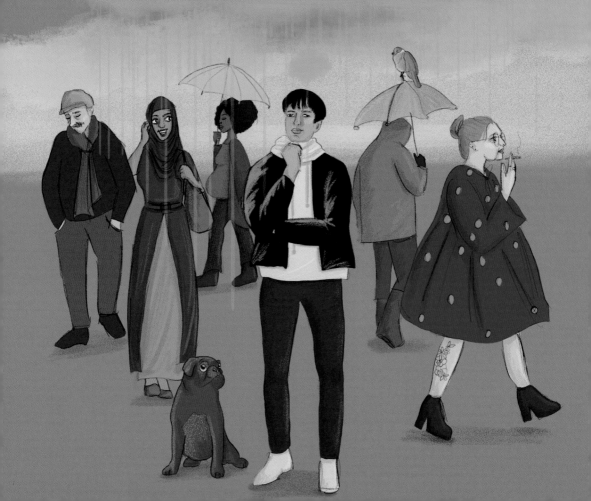

HISTORY OF MENTAL ILLNESS

On the whole, on the wider human scale of history, mental illness is invisible. This could go some way towards explaining why ancient historical explanations of mental disorders often lay in the supernatural or the evil, and were difficult to comprehend. In Mesopotamia, mental illness was believed to have been dealt to humans by the gods. In ancient India, mental disorders represented the supernatural, witches, and sorcery. The Middle Ages saw a great number of different theories in Europe, some intertwined with the idea that this was people's punishment for sin. No wonder mental health is still so stigmatized!

Today we recognize that mental health disorders are related to psychology, but as they're still invisible, we can't always grasp to what extent people around us are affected. Every year one in four of us is affected by poor mental health, so the chances are that you'll either experience it yourself or know someone going through it.

Mental health problems in children ages 3 to 17

in 2017-2018
1 in 5 (21.9%)

in 2020-2021
1 in 4 (23.3%)

Results published by the National Survey of Children's Health

Registered suicides
(in the US)

in 2021
47,646

♀
♂

Data from CDC/National Center for Health Statistics

Suffering from mental illness
(in US)

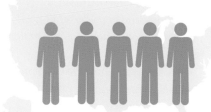

Data from the Centers for Disease Control and Prevention (CDC)

Most common disorders
(in US)

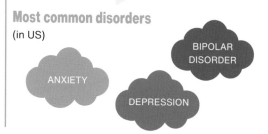

ANXIETY

DEPRESSION

BIPOLAR DISORDER

IS MENTAL ILLNESS JUST A NORMAL PART OF THE HUMAN EXPERIENCE?

Some argue that having poor mental health is just a normal part of the human experience. And we can witness in our language how differently it is treated by people who don't recognize what they can't see. There is an inference that you can "snap out of it," and yet with physical conditions such as cancer or broken bones, such language would never be used.

It's as if mental illness is self-inflicted or made up, and the brain is a different entity from the rest of the body and doesn't suffer. Yet the brain is a part of the body and impacts other bodily functions. Mental health is too integral to ignore and dismiss.

Yes, the stats show that poor mental health is a very common part of the human experience, but that doesn't mean it should be normalized. Just as people can be screened for their physical health—for example, cancer (which one in two of us will get), diabetes, and heart conditions—so mental health screening should also be given weight and importance.

WHAT IS TOXIC POSITIVITY?

While there is space for a positive mental attitude, a sunny disposition, and working through negative thoughts, insisting on positive vibes 100 percent of the time is unrealistic, dismisses negative emotions and poor mental health, and encourages others to mask their pain—sometimes things aren't sunshine and rainbows.

While many people who use these phrases are completely well-meaning, it can feel dismissive to the other person who is trying to communicate pain. Negative emotions are uncomfortable to deal with, but you don't have to try to change their outlook.

Toxic positivity

- "Look on the bright side"
- "It can't be that bad"
- "It'll be fine"
- "It could be worse"
- "You'll get over it"

Helpful positivity + validation

- "This sounds awful! How can I help?"
- "I'm so sorry this is happening"
- "Is there anything you'd like to do today?"
- "I'm here for you if you need to talk"
- "It's okay to feel this way. I love you and am here for you"

SUPPRESSING EMOTIONS

From a young age, we're taught that emotions are irrational, a sign of weakness—particularly the negative ones. We have passed down the idea that we need to have a strong facade of togetherness—that crying is a betrayal of our ability to be self-sufficient, revealing that we're not coping. Gender stereotypes have contributed to a culture where men crying is seen as a betrayal of their toughness. Anger is a much less taboo emotion in men compared to sadness; aggression is seemingly much more expected than crying. There is still this societal embarrassment around crying: around not wanting to admit to ourselves that we may need help, not wanting to be a burden on others, and an ongoing "stiff upper lip" mentality that requires emotions to be dealt with in private.

And then there is shock when seemingly smiley, happy people reveal they have depression or end their lives. Is it any wonder, when we've been told "it can't be that bad, don't cry," and are encouraged to deal with emotions on our own? Just because someone is smiling, it doesn't mean they're happy.

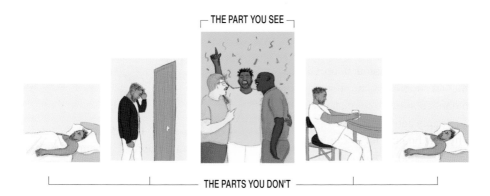

THE PART YOU SEE

THE PARTS YOU DON'T

You don't know what's going on in people's lives, so check in on your friends, including the happy ones.

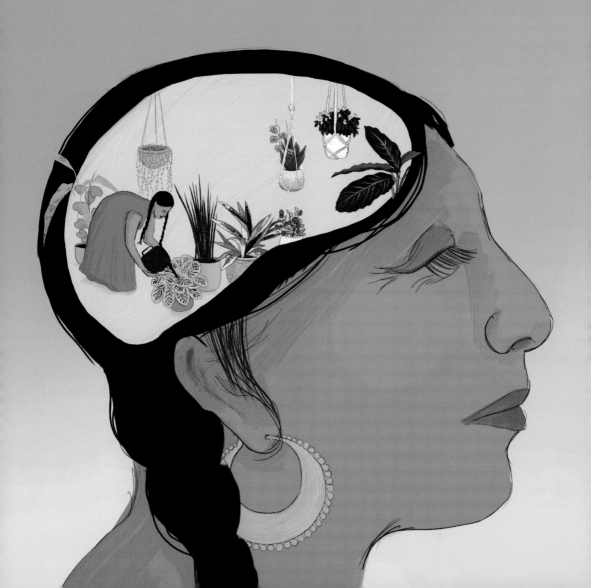

How to maintain good mental health was googled more than ever in 2021. The most searched-for mental health topics were anxiety (36 percent), depression (23 percent), autism (16 percent), Attention Deficit Hyperactivity Disorder (ADHD) (16 percent), and bipolar disorder (8 percent). With that in mind, I am focusing here on anxiety, depression, and the difference between depression and low mood. I will address autism and ADHD later in the book (see page 180).

Low mood is a state of sadness, frustration, and glumness. It varies in severity, and many people experience this as—loosely—bad days. There are thought to be many things that impact our mood, including general health, being active, how much sleep we're getting, what's going on currently in our life, our connections with others, and even the weather. And, at its most severe, low mood can turn into depression.

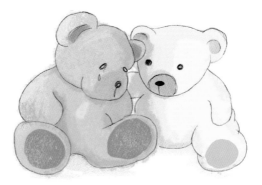

A LOW-MOOD TOOLKIT

1. RECOGNIZE NEGATIVE THOUGHT PATTERNS (SOME BASIC CBT):

A large component of CBT—cognitive behavioral therapy—which is the main form of talking therapy prescribed by doctors, is that our beliefs and (interpretation of our) thoughts can impact our mood, behavior, and feelings. Being aware, recognizing these patterns of thought, and reframing them may be helpful in preventing a spiral. Here are just a few examples . . .

	DESCRIPTION	EXAMPLE	ANTIDOTE
Black-and-white thinking	It's either this or that.	If it's not perfect, it's ruined.	Consider the middle ground, not just extremes.
Mind reading and assumptions	Jumping to conclusions and creating your own narrative about what someone else must be thinking.	He hasn't spoken to me in ages, therefore he hates me.	Ask what people really think.
Crystal-ball gazing	Predicting the result, which can stop us from doing things because we've already "seen" the result and decided there's no point.	I don't have the experience, so I won't go for the job because I know I won't get it.	Remember that you are not a mystic. Your mind is skewed in a negative way for protection, but anything could happen, and it won't necessarily be a negative outcome.

	DESCRIPTION	EXAMPLE	ANTIDOTE
Disqualifying the positive	Focusing solely on the negative, even when there's evidence of positives.	Receiving a compliment on cooking a really nice meal, but discounting it because the potatoes were slightly burnt.	Speak to yourself as you would to a friend—would you only search for negatives? Recognize the positives.
Catastrophizing	A thought spiral that ruminates on worst case scenarios and makes the very worst of situations.	What if X happens?	Step back and remind yourself of the most probable scenario and also play out the "what ifs"—figure out what steps you would take; we can never actually answer all of the "what ifs."
"Should" statements	"Shoulds" are specifically based on guilt or shame. When things revolve around what you *should* do, it is an immediate put-down that you're not doing something well enough or are not where you should be.	I should be more successful by now.	Work out your values and use them as motivation, instead of shame and guilt.
Emotional reasoning	Accepting emotions as evidence for the truth.	I feel worthless, so I am worthless.	Remember that feelings are not facts, and they are not the whole truth.

2. REACH OUT TO LOVED ONES WHO HAVE A LOT OF EMPATHY, OR GENERALLY CAN CHEER YOU UP:

Human beings need others, and we want to be seen. Having someone who can just listen or cheer us up in a way that doesn't diminish what we're feeling can make the world of difference. Just try to check if they have the capacity to listen before emotionally dumping on them!

3. TAKE ONE STEP AT A TIME:

When everything feels too tough, just focus on the first step, even if it's only willing yourself to get out of bed.

4. CREATE A MENTAL HEALTH FIRST-AID KIT:

Fill a box with things that you know lift your mood or perk you up—music playlists, cards from people who love you, photos of cherished memories and loved ones, vitamins, cute dog pictures, fidget toys, tiny pumpkins, chocolates, whatever things you enjoy that make you feel good.

5. THERAPY:

If you have the means, or have access to some free support, good therapists help many people. This solution doesn't suit everyone, but sometimes it's a case of trying a different therapist or form of therapy to suit your needs.

Low mood and depression have different severities, so while these tips may help some, others may need further professional advice. People and mental illnesses are varied and different.

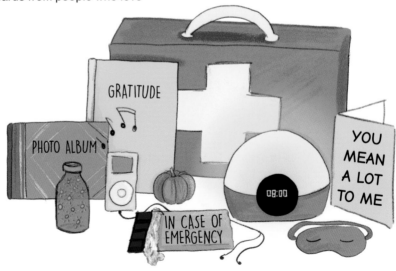

MY OWN EXPERIENCE
OF DEPRESSION & SUICIDAL IDEATION

I wanted to keep myself largely out of this book, but this part feels too hard to reduce to some bullet points, and I thought a personal tale would give a little more insight. While I find the suggestions given helpful on a bad day, at my most depressed I would have had no interest in any of them . . .

Just after university, after a series of losses and setbacks, I experienced a nine-month-long depression interspersed with regular suicidal thoughts, often about jumping in front of a train on my way to an internship I was doing at the time. I'd glaze over for the train ride, have tears running down my face while walking to the internship, and then plaster on a smile and go about my day, until I came home later and was left with my thoughts. I listened to a lot of Lana del Rey songs while sobbing silently in the bath. I didn't want other people to know, but instead of being sad, I was outwardly angry and snappy towards those who were close to me.

When a well-meaning family member begged to know what was wrong, I told them I felt suicidal and they said they didn't understand, it couldn't be that bad, and they thought it was selfish of me. I felt guilty. A friend said it wasn't that bad because I hadn't actually done anything. I felt like my own experience didn't count and maybe I should escalate things, in order for people to take my pain seriously.

I met up with a childhood friend who was battling depression at the same time as me, and we talked and listened and related to each other. It was a breath of fresh air as we bonded so much more, and laughed and joked about how depressed we were. When you're experiencing something that bad, I think it helps to find someone who understands, and with whom you can laugh about it. We would set small goals for ourselves for the next time we would meet up. Usually around mental health baby steps, and would report and celebrate our small wins or discuss our relapses.

There were a few things that got me through those bad days, and I'd love to share them with you here—however, I recognize our brains are unique and complex and what might work for me might not for someone else:

THINGS THAT HELPED ME PERSONALLY AT THE TIME, AND ON CURRENT BAD DAYS

- Having people who really cared and would check in, even if they didn't know what to say.

- Having someone who really "gets it" and can listen: having people who checked in was much needed and appreciated, but the person who completely understood made me feel less alone in my struggle.

- Having a responsibility (the internship) and being a people-pleaser: I'm afraid to say that I didn't want to let my bosses down, so I forced myself to get there somehow. The work was pleasant and distracting enough.

- Very long, sad playlists: to release the emotions.

- One step at a time: "Okay, now get out of bed." I can't stress how that alone required so much effort. If you know, you know.

- Time: this particular period did start with a series of losses, so it was situational and time helped to make those losses less all-consuming.

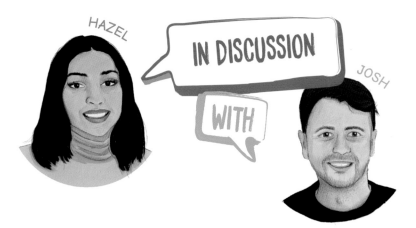

HAZEL

IN DISCUSSION WITH

JOSH

With anxiety being so prevalent in modern-day society, I interviewed Joshua Fletcher, a.k.a. Anxiety Josh, a psychotherapist specializing in anxiety and the host of The Panic Pod, a podcast covering all things related to anxiety and panic recovery. He is also the author of three bestselling books: *Anxiety: Panicking About Panic, Anxiety: Practical About Panic,* and (with Dean Stott) *Untangle Your Anxiety: A Guide to Overcoming an Anxiety Disorder by Two People Who Have Been Through It.*

What does anxiety feel like? How does it manifest itself?

Anxiety manifests itself in thoughts, feelings, and sensations.

1. You know it's an anxious thought because it'll begin with "What if": "What if this happens?" That's 90 percent acute anxiety. Then you've got "I should": "I should be productive." And "I can't": "I can't do this. There's no point in even trying." Pretty much all anxiety starts with those three precursors.

2. Feelings can range between nervousness, dread, doom, a horrible sense of foreboding, terror, fright, panic, and fear. It's like a pick 'n' mix box.

3. Then you've got sensations: physical sensations, like a tight chest or heart palpitations. One of the most common but unspoken ones is derealization or dissociation, where you feel detached from yourself—it's called depersonalization as well—so you feel detached from your body. Sweating, butterflies in your stomach, muscle tension, strange symptoms like eye floaters, itchy skin, dizziness,

lightheadedness, "I can't catch my breath," or "I feel like I need to go to the bathroom."

There are two different types of anxiety. You've got your conventional outwards anxiety that everyone can relate to: first day, job interview, doctor's appointment. And then you've got disordered anxiety, the inwards stuff: nasty intrusive thoughts about harm, thoughts about panicking, panic attacks, being convinced you're dying, obsessive compulsive disorder (OCD), and clinical trauma, as in post-traumatic stress disorder (PTSD).

Are there any coping mechanisms that can help with anxiety attacks if you find yourself in the midst of one?

Yeah, you don't do anything. This is the whole myth of panic attacks and anxiety. No one's ever died from an anxiety/panic attack. They're not dangerous; they're just extremely uncomfortable.

If I start breathing into a brown paper bag and then I calm down, I don't get the credit for tolerating my anxiety—the bag does!

If I 100 percent rely on my partner to calm me down from panic attacks, all my brain learns is that I can't tolerate it: you have to have your partner to help. And suddenly you're getting safety behaviors.

So you remind yourself, "Hey, this is just adrenaline and cortisol, it's in your bloodstream now—it will pass. It's not going to hurt you. Try not to avoid it, and pat yourself on the back when it passes."

You've just taught the brain: "Look, I can tolerate this huge level of discomfort." Panic attacks don't last forever—you're not going to go crazy. And those symptoms, that's just adrenaline.

If I go into a room and my threat response is saying to me, "What if I shit myself and I can't get to the bathroom?", then I go, "Just in case, I'll hang around near the bathroom." What I've signaled to my brain is that that irrational thought is actually dangerous, so now every time I socialize, I'll always be near the bathroom, because I've just started a new anxious behavior.

Is there anything more long-term or ongoing that you would recommend, to improve your relationship with yourself and your anxiety?

Self-compassion is really important. If you take anyone with social anxiety and hear their thoughts out loud and talking, it's like a constant commentary of self-criticism.

Your anxiety is because of your involuntary nervous system, which is split into two: your sympathetic nervous system,

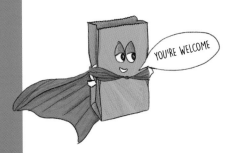

YOU'RE WELCOME

which causes stress, panic, and anxiety, and your parasympathetic nervous system—the rest-and-digest part: laughing, getting a massage, sleeping enough.

A lot of people think it's all work, work, work. But then if you don't balance it out with parasympathetic nervous system stuff, you end up having burnout. You know you've got an imbalance when you wake up with dread every morning, or you go to bed with dread, or you're just ruminating for hours.

Are there any common misconceptions or myths that people have about anxiety?
You've got the tropes—like OCD is not an adjective, it's a really severe disorder.

Panic attacks are not like those you see on Netflix. They're mostly freezing responses. "Anxiety condition" is now called a "fight, flight, freeze, and fawn response." We've all heard of "fight or flight." The freeze response is what a lot of people with social anxiety do—maybe I want to run away, but I can't, so I just freeze in place. Fawning is what people pleasers, or people who've been through trauma and social anxiety, do. When they're anxious they want to make sure their boss, or their partner, isn't unhappy with them. And that's all part of anxiety—the same anxious response. The only difference is the threat. Anxiety is many different things and it can present itself in many different ways. ■

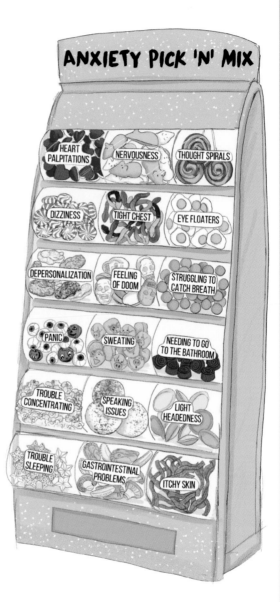

WHAT IS SELF-CARE?

"Self-care" has become synonymous with bath bombs, yoga retreats, and face masks—basically, fancy products for when you want to "treat yourself. While there is space for that, the original meaning of self-care has been washed out, and it's become something you can only have access to if you have the money to afford luxuries. Self-care, like many other wellbeing practices—such as yoga, which actually has roots in a humble spiritual practice rather than showing off your flexibility—has become monetized by companies seeking to increase wealth by jumping on these trends. Self-care is remembering the self. It's looking after your basic needs. It can be quite dull at times. It can be whatever you need it to be! It can absolutely be a bath with candles if you want, but it's also closing your email after 6 p.m. or moving your body or eating the broccoli or leaving a job where the boss bullies you.

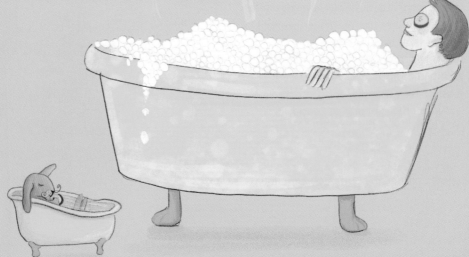

THE ORIGINS OF SELF-CARE

While "self-care" may be a term from a recent vernacular, the concept has been around for a while. The ancient Greek philosopher Socrates allegedly asked, "Are you not ashamed for devoting all your care to increasing your wealth, reputation, and honors, while not caring or even considering your reason, truth, and constant improvement of the soul?" At that point in time he was speaking about working on self-improvement and soul work, which would have included looking after one's mental, physical, and spiritual health.

Self-care was later encouraged by those in the medical professions—prescribing healthy lifestyles and taking your health into your own hands. It was the women's rights and civil rights movements that started advocating self-care as a political act for the marginalized.

African American writer-activist Audre Lorde, when dying of cancer, spoke of self-care as a response to a society that oppresses and does not care for everyone equally. As she wrote in *A Burst of Light* in 1988, "Caring for myself is not self-indulgence, it is self-preservation, and that is an act of political warfare." She also examined the difference between stretching and overextending oneself—a message that is still relevant today. It's not about not working hard for what you believe in. It's about resisting a society that celebrates and glamorizes hustle, grind, and over-exertion of the self as a marker of worth.

We also need to recognize community care as being important in society, helping others when the government fails us. It's marching for the rights of others; it's speaking out against hate; it's helping out a neighbor, being there for a friend, volunteering; it's supporting local businesses. But rest and revolution go together. Many who dedicate time to helping and caring for others feel too guilty to make time for themselves, yet they are arguably the ones who need to do so the most. Self-care is not selfish.

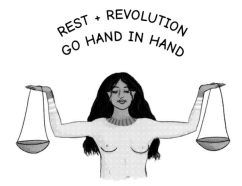

REST + REVOLUTION GO HAND IN HAND

SELF-CARE CAN BE MANY THINGS

LISTEN TO MUSIC

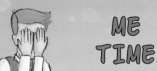

HAVE A GOOD CRY

ME TIME

EAT NUTRITIOUS FOOD

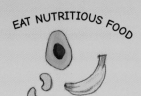

MEDITATE

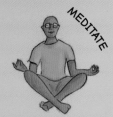

READ

SLEEEEEEEP

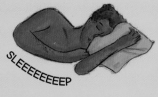

MASTURBATE

EXERCISE

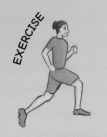

GET SOME SUN

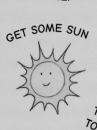

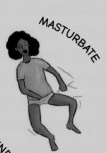

TALK KINDLY TO YOURSELF

YOGA

THERAPY

EAT COMFORT FOOD

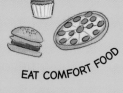

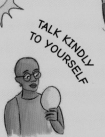

GET TO KNOW YOUR BODY

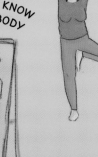

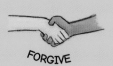

FORGIVE

WALK MINDFULLY

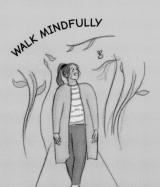

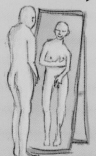

REDUCE TIME WITH TOXIC PEOPLE

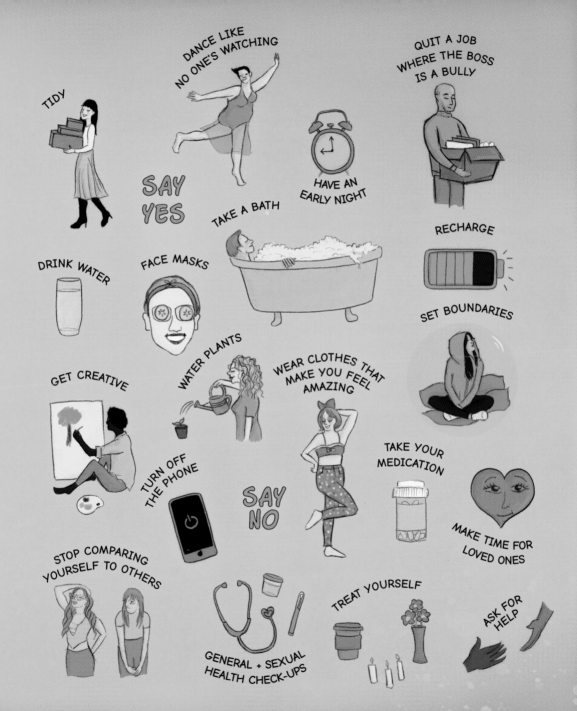

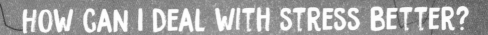

Classical theory suggests that we evolved stress responses to allow for short-term immediate benefits, such as fight or flight, through the sympathetic nervous system, which speeds up your heart rate in a real or perceived emergency. While nowadays most of us aren't fleeing from lions, tigers, or bears, we still have stresses in our lives, such as deadlines, major life episodes, and the effects of world events. Whatever your personal stresses are, they have the same effect.

During those stressful situations, our bodies go into survival mode, needing energy for muscles, so glucose and fat are moved to the bloodstream while our heart rate and breathing intensify. Our senses are sharpened, too. Other bodily functions are put on pause or decrease, including bodily repairs, the immune system, sex drive, and more. While this is beneficial for immediate danger, if it becomes constant and chronic, stress can have negative long-term impacts on many aspects of our lives, including sleep, the reproductive system, libido, and aging, and can cause heart disease, diabetes, and strokes.

WHERE WE HOLD STRESS IN THE BODY

Stress can store itself in the body without you even realizing. The body and mind are so intrinsically linked. Tight muscles can be a sign of repressed emotions or stress. Perhaps you're clenching your jaw muscles or feel like you have the weight of the world on your shoulders. Even that phrase speaks of the tension you're feeling, both mentally and physically.

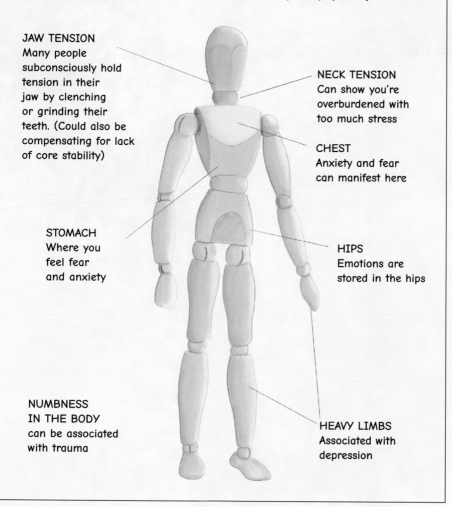

JAW TENSION
Many people subconsciously hold tension in their jaw by clenching or grinding their teeth. (Could also be compensating for lack of core stability)

NECK TENSION
Can show you're overburdened with too much stress

CHEST
Anxiety and fear can manifest here

STOMACH
Where you feel fear and anxiety

HIPS
Emotions are stored in the hips

NUMBNESS IN THE BODY
can be associated with trauma

HEAVY LIMBS
Associated with depression

Yin yoga offers long, deep stretches which can tackle that physical tension. Its philosophy is rooted in the concept of yin and yang *chi*, or vital energy— yin embraces the cooling, restorative elements, as opposed to yang yoga, which is more active. Because of this letting go, and holding poses for longer, it's not uncommon for emotions to crop up, as physical tension is often linked to mental tension. In this respect, yin yoga can be a tough practice, especially for those who are uncomfortable being left with their own thoughts, because in a very yang society we are not often left in long moments of stillness.

WHY DO I NEED TO RELEARN BREATHING?

Stress can also be tackled using something so simple—our breathing. It's something we do naturally, although most of us aren't breathing deeply. It has numerous benefits, including regulating stress, slowing the heart rate, and lowering our blood pressure. There are many techniques, one of which is provided on page 121.

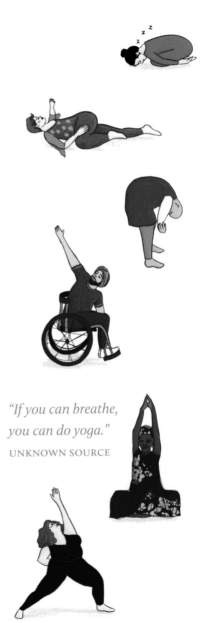

"If you can breathe, you can do yoga."
UNKNOWN SOURCE

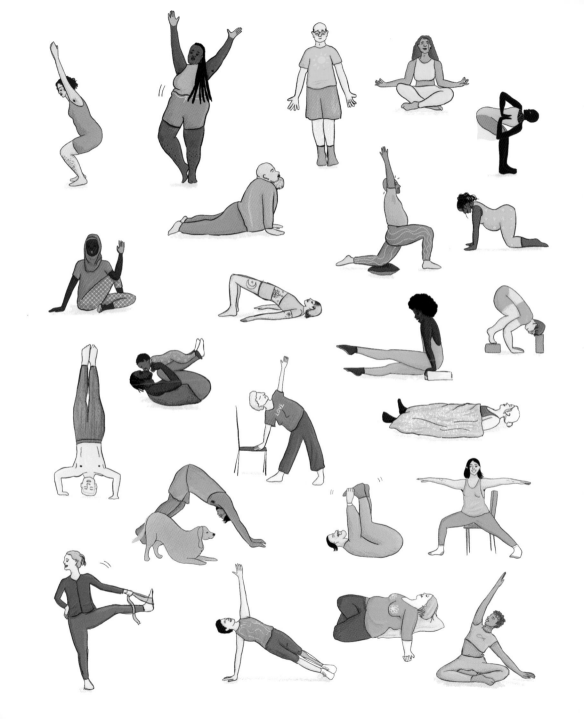

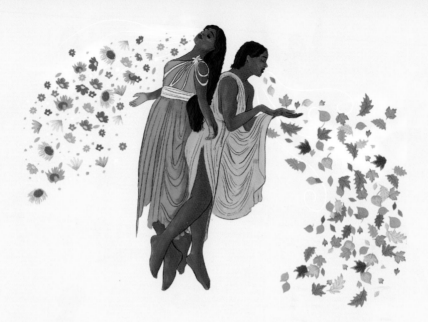

BREATHING

Deep breathing activates the parasympathetic nervous system—a network of nerves that relaxes your body—and the vagus nerve, which affects mood and heart rate, and sends more oxygen to your brain.

We often forget to breathe deeply, and shallow breathing can stress us out more. A deeper breath can help regulate the body and control anger and anxiety in the moment.

TRY THIS EXERCISE

Sit upright but comfortably, or lie on your back.

Close your eyes and notice how you're breathing. You can put one hand on your chest and the other on your stomach.

Start to deepen your breath by inhaling through the nose and focusing the breath down so your stomach moves outwards. Then exhale so the stomach falls back into place.

REVISIT THIS PAGE WHEN YOU NEED A MOMENT.
TRACE YOUR FINGER ALONG THE ARROWS AND BREATHE.

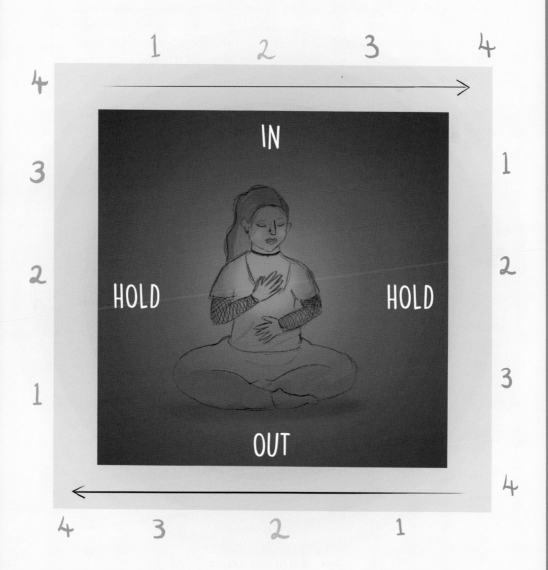

STRESS CYCLES

In busy, present-day life, many people find themselves in a constant, ongoing state of stress. Our bodies don't differentiate between stresses, and they still go through the same physiological processes, whether we're running from a lion or dealing with a demanding boss. When running from a lion, there is a clear indication when the stress has ended—after running, our bodies know to return to homeostasis (our baseline state). Drs. Emily and Amelia Nagoski argue that, unlike running from a lion, when dealing with ongoing stresses we don't manage to close our stress cycles, and we need to intervene to signal to our body that it is safe by speaking its language—body language.

They propose some practical ways to close the stress cycle, including exercise or moving the body, crying, laughter, and affection, such as a long hug or kiss with a close one.

A NOTE ON EXERCISE

You don't have to be in the gym if that's not your thing!

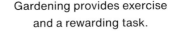

Aerobic exercise can boost endorphins—hormones that your body produces to relieve pain and make you feel good.

Boxing and sparring can be great ways to release anger and stress. Strolling in nature can provide a multisensory experience.

Gardening provides exercise and a rewarding task.

Don't forget about NEAT exercise: it all counts. NEAT stands for "non-exercise activity thermogenesis" and refers to any energy used on activities that aren't traditionally classed as exercise: anything active that you do in your daily life, such as cooking, carrying the groceries, taking the stairs, DIY projects, or playing with a pet.

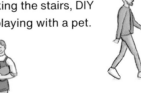

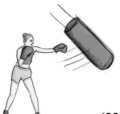

CONTROL

While the body provides keys to releasing stress, there are mental hacks that may be of help, too. If you feel like you worry about every little thing and it's affecting you in a negative way, one thought that was proposed by the Stoics could help: you should only concern yourself with what you can control. When you realize there are things that are out of your control, then there is no point in worrying about them because there's nothing you can do to change them.

For example, the bus being stuck in traffic is out of your control, so it is not useful to worry about it while you're on that bus. Death is inevitable, so fearing death every day is going to lead to a lifetime of pointless worry. Consider this concept and how you can use it to free your mind. Of course, this is much easier said than done, but in a moment of stress, try to think about whether or not this is something you can control.

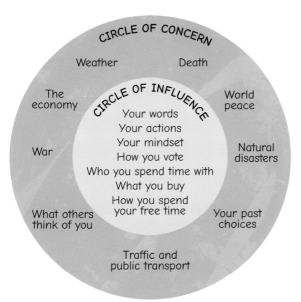

CIRCLE OF CONCERN

Weather   Death

The economy   World peace

CIRCLE OF INFLUENCE
Your words
Your actions
Your mindset
How you vote
Who you spend time with
What you buy
How you spend your free time

War   Natural disasters

What others think of you   Your past choices

Traffic and public transport

"If there is no solution to the problem then don't waste time worrying about it. If there is a solution to the problem then don't waste time worrying about it."

THE 14TH DALAI LAMA

HOW DO I COPE WITH GRIEF?

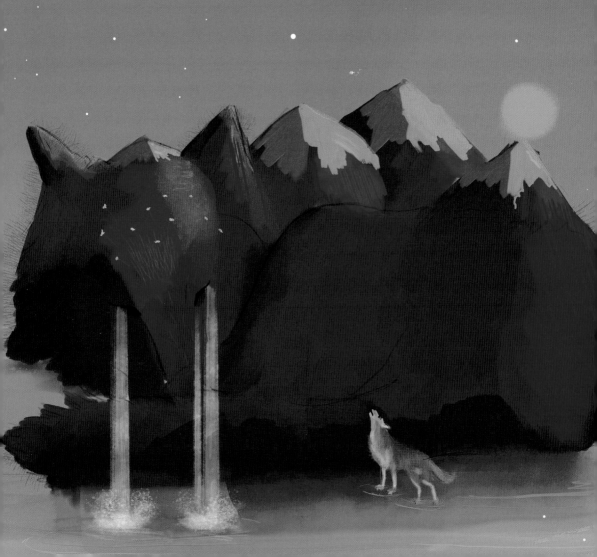

When you think about grief and how to cope, perhaps you conjure up the well-known five stages of grief: denial, anger, bargaining, depression, and acceptance. Although this is a now well-popularized manual for the journey of grief generally, the studies these stages derived from, conducted by the psychiatrist Elisabeth Kübler-Ross, were based solely on patients coming to terms with their terminal diagnoses. In reality, everyone's grief journey is different, nuanced, non-linear, and may come in waves of different emotions and intensities.

GRIEF RITUALS IN DIFFERENT CULTURES

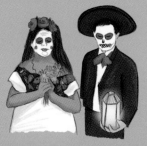

Victorians wore all-black as an outward display of grief and had a whole etiquette manual, which detailed appropriate materials to wear.

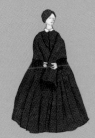

Famadihana or the "turning of the bones" is a Madagascan funerary tradition, where once every 5–7 years, family visit the ancestral crypt where bodies wrapped in cloth are exhumed and sprayed with wine and perfume. Some share family news with the deceased. Others reminisce and tell stories.

Mexico's Day of the Dead has a joyful, celebratory feel and encourages people to talk about and remember their loved ones who have died.

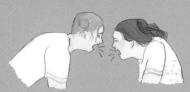

Throughout various cultures, including those of ancient Celts and indigenous peoples of Africa, Asia, South America, and Australia, emotion is performed ceremoniously through a "death wail" or keening.

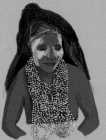

Specific mourning attire is also worn in Papua New Guinea. A widow may wear lots of necklaces made from seeds. One by one, the necklaces are removed, until the last one is taken off at a ceremony, which ends the mourning period.

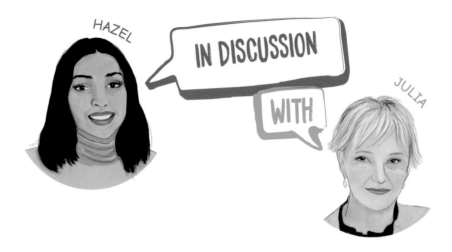

HAZEL

IN DISCUSSION WITH

JULIA

There is no one way to grieve. Different cultures have different customs and ways of expressing grief and mourning the loss of loved ones, and even within those cultures, grief can vary in each person. What's more, as I learned when the psychotherapist Julia Samuel introduced me to the concept of "living losses," grief does not only occur with a literal death. Here is our discussion on dealing with grief.

Why is grief so taboo or even awkward at times?

There is a kind of magical thinking that we have, which is, "If I think or talk about death, it will in some way hasten my death, or the death of people that I love. And so if I don't think about it, if I don't talk about it, then perhaps it's not going to happen to me." We also fear the unknown, and what we don't have control over. So it is a sort of defense mechanism, a way of dealing with the unknown and our powerlessness.

The other thing that is often actually under-discussed is that we may talk about the fact that we're going to die, or that the people we love will die, but we never talk about the fact that we're going to be bereaved. And what grief actually feels like. So we don't talk to the people that we love about our own death and dying. And so there's no preparation.

We've been referring to grief in terms of death, but what else, in your experience, do you find people are grieving? Can you tell us more about the concept of living losses?

Living losses can be losses from a divorce or separation, they can occur from moving country, losing a job, getting a health diagnosis. We can be very reductionist about the external event—e.g., you move house, and that's you sorted. But even when these are things we wanted, like getting married, or committing to a partner, or having children, the adaptation process is experienced like grief, but isn't legitimized or acknowledged.

So what emotions are natural in that process?

Grief is a very messy, chaotic process. You can have feelings of sadness and fury, and terror and confusion, and numbness and despair, stuckness—and that affects all your physiological processes: sleeping, not sleeping, eating, not eating. Grief often shoots through your body like fear, because life as you know it is irrevocably changed. Pain is the agent of change; pain is the thing that forces us to face this new reality that we didn't want, that we didn't choose.

And so when we have that feeling, it is the things we do that support us to allow it to come through our system, rather than the mechanisms that we use to block it, which do us harm. Allowing it to come through our system is how we adapt and change and even grow through it.

In those early stages, can escapism be healthy? Is it better to push pain away a bit, just to get through the days?

We can't make ourselves not feel particular feelings, but I think we can support ourselves through them. Distraction, denial, busyness, painting, watching movies, or whatever it is you do, can give you a break from the pain.

It is a dual process of loss orientation, where you may grieve and feel pain; and restoration orientation, where you have hope for the future, where you make plans, where you get on with your day, have a break from the pain, distract yourself. It's the movement between the two that is the process.

Is there any way that you'd recommend starting the healing process?

I think one key thing is support—the love and connection that you receive at the time of the loss is what makes the difference. The love and connection of others, but also your relationship with yourself: being compassionate to yourself and turning to yourself with warmth, not criticism. We often attack ourselves when we're grieving and that's extremely unhealthy: the guilt, ruminating and "what ifs," and the belief that "I'm doing this badly—I'm failing even at grieving."

How can you be there for someone who is grieving? Any dos and don'ts?

Listen, show up, don't turn away, don't cross the street. Offer practical help, whether that's food or taking the children, going for a walk with them. The key thing, if you're a close friend, is to be there for the long haul. People are often there at the beginning, in the first few months, but then they will get back to their lives.

I suppose it's not linear and time-dependent, how long you're supposed to grieve? Does it ever go away?

Society is a bit mechanistic—if it's for grandparents, I'll give you three months. If it's for a parent, six months to a year. But the level of the loss is equal to the level of the love and the emotional significance of the person in your life. We don't get over grief—we learn to accommodate, adapt, grow through it, and live with it.

It is an iterative process that takes time. The intensity, and those waves that hit people, depend on the relationship with the person, the circumstances of the death, the support you have.

One of the things I talk to clients about is *chronos* time and *kairos* time. *Chronos* time is chronological time, the twenty-four-hour clock, and so on; and *kairos* time is felt time—time that we experience, our internal adaptation process. For grief, it's *kairos* time.

The love for the person you're grieving never dies. It's not about forgetting and moving on, but remembering and loving the person who's died or left your life, while you psychologically adjust to the absence of their presence. ■

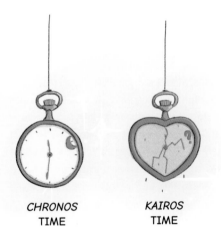

CHRONOS
TIME

KAIROS
TIME

WHY CAN'T I FIND HAPPINESS?

We are all searching for happiness. But what if we're searching for the wrong thing? Perhaps you find yourself saying, "I need X to be happy" or "I'll be happy when . . ." and then when you achieve or get X, the happiness doesn't last all that long.

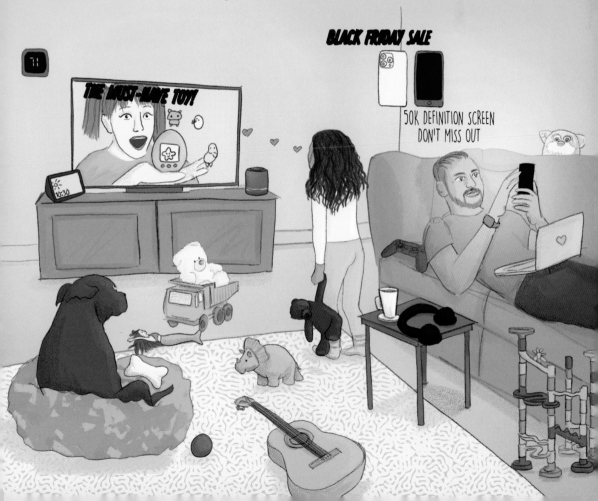

WHY WE CAN'T CONSTANTLY BE HAPPY

You're not broken—it's how we are wired. Happiness is a temporary arousing emotion, so we can't constantly be experiencing it. When we experience a consistent positive life change (for example, a promotion, or a bigger home, or dating an amazing partner), the elation and excitement that come with novelty wear off as we become used to this improved life change. It becomes our normal and we may then find ourselves searching for the next thing that will make us happy.

THIS SHOULD BRING HAPPINESS

The economy thrives on people spending money, so having a society that can convince people they need to buy things to make them happy is beneficial. Next time you look at ads, notice how many are targeted at convincing you how much better your life would be if you had that product; if you had that perfume, how many more admirers you'd have; if you had that car, how many people would envy you; if you didn't have that smartphone, what a lot of features you would be missing out on. It's clever marketing, targeting our insecurities and our quest for happiness. Be aware of what's being sold to you.

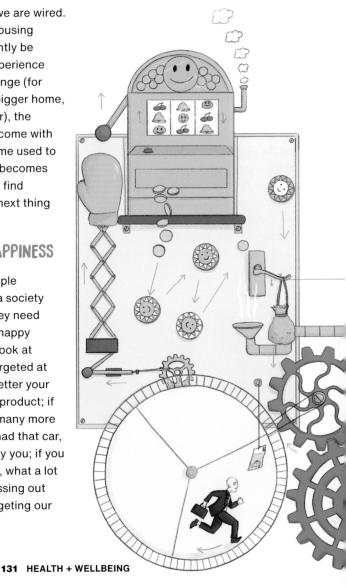

IMPACT BIAS

Unfortunately, we have an impact bias, where we overestimate the intensity of emotions, so we often think things will bring more happiness than they do. Unlike other animals, we are able to imagine how a situation will pan out, so if we're invisioning the joy we'll get from a certain trip, and yet the weather wasn't great, the food gave us an upset stomach, and the plane was delayed, it sets us up for disappointment. It works the other way, too. A break-up that we think we will never get over will heal with time and the emotions won't feel as awful. This mechanism means that we often overestimate what things will bring us joy.

DRIP-FEEDING HAPPINESS AND DOPAMINE

If we're setting ourselves up to fail, by overhyping what things will be like in the future, then how can we combat this? It goes back to trying to find joy in those little moments, being present, and focusing on the *now*. Perhaps you've blocked them out or aren't paying attention to them, but today try writing down all the little tiny things that you've enjoyed. These can bring happiness just as much as the big vacations and achievements.

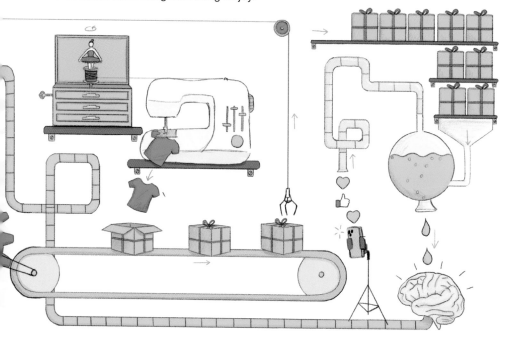

IT'S THE SMALL THINGS IN LIFE

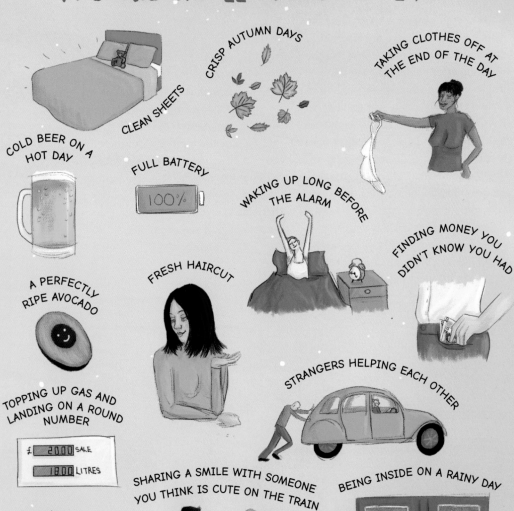

CLEAN SHEETS

CRISP AUTUMN DAYS

TAKING CLOTHES OFF AT THE END OF THE DAY

COLD BEER ON A HOT DAY

FULL BATTERY

WAKING UP LONG BEFORE THE ALARM

FINDING MONEY YOU DIDN'T KNOW YOU HAD

A PERFECTLY RIPE AVOCADO

FRESH HAIRCUT

STRANGERS HELPING EACH OTHER

TOPPING UP GAS AND LANDING ON A ROUND NUMBER

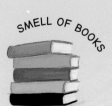

£ 20.00 SALE

18.00 LITRES

SHARING A SMILE WITH SOMEONE YOU THINK IS CUTE ON THE TRAIN

BEING INSIDE ON A RAINY DAY

SMELL OF BOOKS

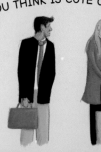

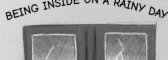

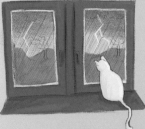

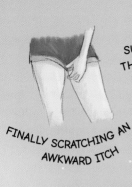

FINALLY SCRATCHING AN AWKWARD ITCH

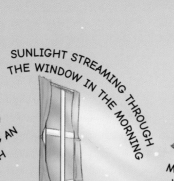

SUNLIGHT STREAMING THROUGH THE WINDOW IN THE MORNING

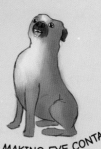
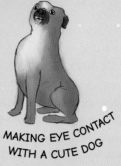

MAKING EYE CONTACT WITH A CUTE DOG

AN EMPTY INBOX

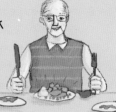

WHEN YOUR FOOD LOOKS BETTER THAN EVERYONE ELSE'S

WALKING BEHIND SOMEONE WHO SMELLS REALLY GOOD

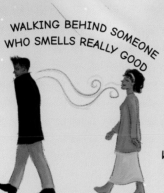

PUTTING ON A SCREEN PROTECTOR WITH NO BUBBLES

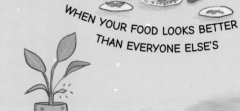

WHEN YOUR HOUSEPLANT GROWS A NEW LEAF

EXTRA SHARP PENCILS

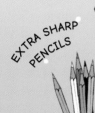

REORGANIZING SHELVES

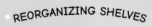
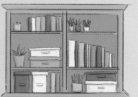
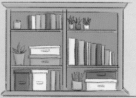

WAVES LAPPING ON THE SHORE

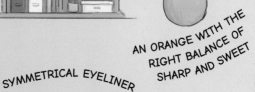

DRESSES WITH POCKETS

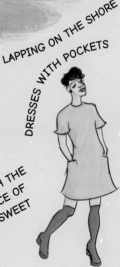

THE COLD SIDE OF THE PILLOW

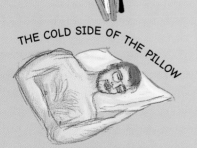

AN ORANGE WITH THE RIGHT BALANCE OF SHARP AND SWEET

SYMMETRICAL EYELINER

THE WORLD HAPPINESS REPORT

In 2020, for the first time, the Gallup World Poll decided to ask participants about balance and harmony. Researchers found that in seven Western nations people defined happiness as "psychological balance and harmony." This was echoed in a more extensive follow-up study which also observed that "inner harmony" was one of the most prominent definitions of happiness.

So perhaps if you're not feeling the happiness you're searching for, shifting the focus to contentment—a positive yet low-arousal feeling—could help. Practicing gratitude, by listing all the things you cherish in life, can help reframe. One final piece of advice is to work out your values and what matters to you, in order to use these bits of wisdom to have a more fulfilling life. A diagram that demonstrates this well is the one below, which is based on diagrams created by Marc Winn and Andrés Zuzunaga.

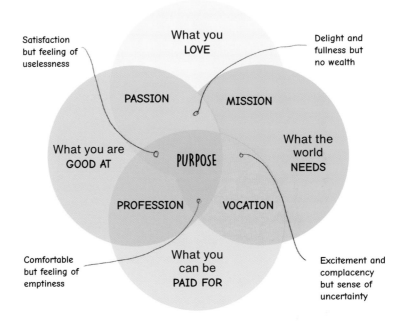

Satisfaction but feeling of uselessness

What you LOVE

Delight and fullness but no wealth

PASSION

MISSION

What you are GOOD AT

PURPOSE

What the world NEEDS

PROFESSION

VOCATION

Comfortable but feeling of emptiness

What you can be PAID FOR

Excitement and complacency but sense of uncertainty

HOW DOES MINDFULNESS WORK?

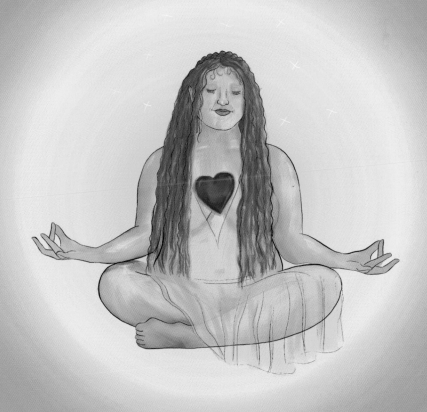

Mindfulness has become a bit of a flowery buzzword, yet it is based on concepts that everyone can benefit from. In this busy, tech-reliant world, with notifications pinging, our brains flit from one thought to another.

Many of us are privileged to live in a world of instant gratification, with food being readily available and streaming sites offering thousands of films, TV series, podcasts, and music playlists to entertain us.

According to multiple studies, including the one discussed on the opposite page, this bombardment of choice is making us less happy, rather than more.

With our brains constantly on the go, always occupied, we can easily turn to autopilot mode for many things, including eating, breathing, and walking.

Mindfulness is about bringing attention back to yourself, your body, and your actions in the present moment.

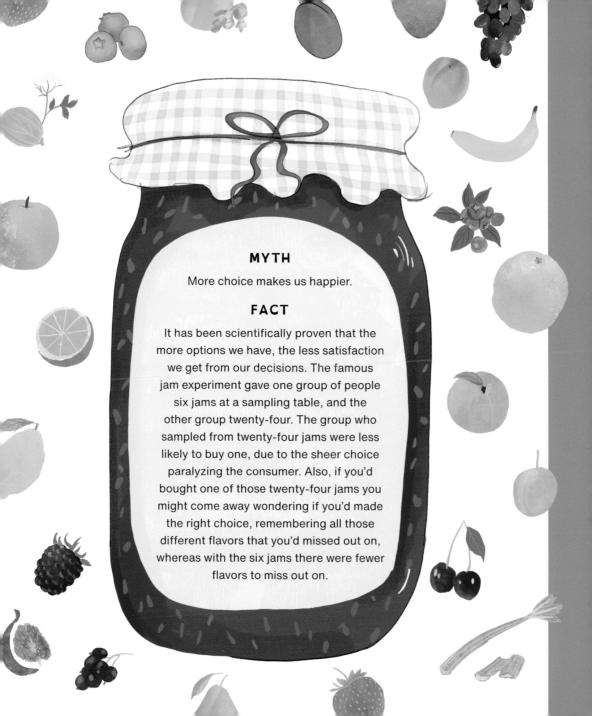

MYTH

More choice makes us happier.

FACT

It has been scientifically proven that the more options we have, the less satisfaction we get from our decisions. The famous jam experiment gave one group of people six jams at a sampling table, and the other group twenty-four. The group who sampled from twenty-four jams were less likely to buy one, due to the sheer choice paralyzing the consumer. Also, if you'd bought one of those twenty-four jams you might come away wondering if you'd made the right choice, remembering all those different flavors that you'd missed out on, whereas with the six jams there were fewer flavors to miss out on.

ESCAPING AUTOPILOT

We've come to glorify hustle culture and productivity, which has brought about the seemingly more productive multitasking, but contrary to how it sounds, multitasking is not necessarily more productive as the brain has to flit from one task to another and spends energy refocusing each time.

For example, it is not uncommon to eat food while doing something else, without really paying attention.

TRY THIS EXERCISE

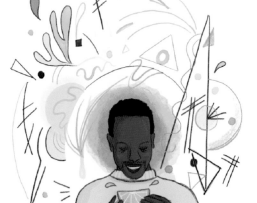

Pick a piece of food that you enjoy (maybe a juicy fruit) and eat it slowly, noticing the look, feel, smell, and taste of it.

Take a few moments to appreciate the food and nothing else: just you and the food.

By just focusing on eating, you are more in tune with your bodily cues, know when you're full, can be more appreciative of what you're eating, and can find more joy in the vast variety of food available to us.

This exercise can also work with walking. When you're out and about, focus on three things you can see, smell, hear, and feel to ground you in the moment.

DON'T BELIEVE EVERYTHING YOU THINK

One useful reflection is that just because a thought feels familiar and true it doesn't mean that it is. As discussed earlier in the low-mood toolkit (see page 105), our thoughts can be incredibly self-critical.

TRY THIS EXERCISE

Close your eyes.

Imagine that each thought that comes into your head is written on a balloon.

Imagine holding each one, reading it, observing it without judgement, then letting go of it.

By viewing your thoughts as physical objects, you can more easily separate yourself from them and acknowledge them for what they are: thoughts, not necessarily truths.

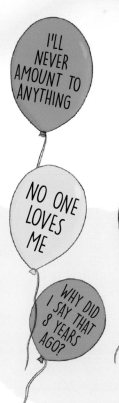
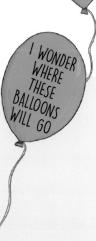

BODY SCAN MEDITATION

A body scan meditation can bring awareness to every part of your body, and make you aware of any tension you may be holding and help you to let it go.

For some people a guided body scan can be helpful and quite hypnotic, once you've found a voice that you enjoy listening to.

TRY THIS EXERCISE

Lie flat on your back, arms by your side and legs parted a little. Gradually begin to draw your focus to your body, what you feel, how your surroundings feel, your breath.

Then, bit by bit, draw your attention up your body. Start with your toes, notice how they feel. Breathe and let them relax. Taking your time, move your attention up to your ankles, calves, thighs, hips, and so on until you reach the crown of your head and have brought awareness to your whole body.

draw your attention to your hands and allow them to completely relax

These are just a few techniques to calm the mind and connect yourself to your body. But mindfulness is more than simply coping mechanisms. Working on mindfulness exercises can also influence how we bring awareness to ourselves and our actions in day-to-day life—responding more than reacting;

being present in our actions; and appreciating our food.

It's also important to note that some people spend their whole lives trying to be mindful. Don't be discouraged—it takes a lot of practice and doesn't have to happen all at once.

IS MY PERIOD NORMAL?

Cultures vary drastically all over the world, but one thing that remains constant in many societies is the misogynistic view that periods are unclean and need to be hidden. It's clear from the fact that there are so many euphemisms used globally to this day instead of the word "period." Not using that word makes the thing itself more taboo.

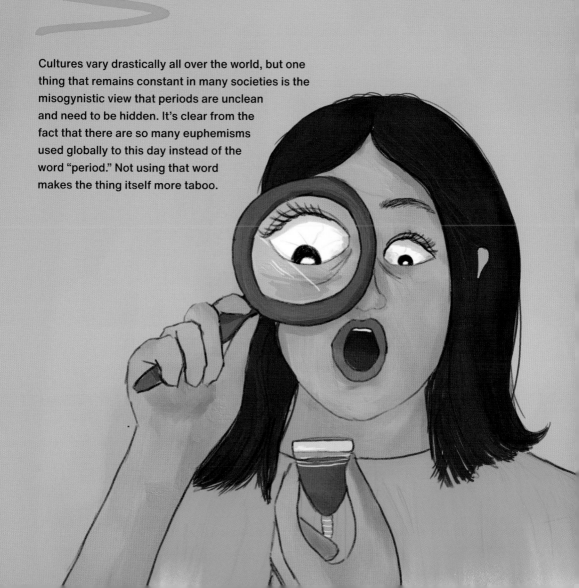

The mystery is further ingrained by separating classes into boys and girls at school and teaching only girls about periods. Menstruation then morphs into mysterious, inexplicable "women's matters" that become hard to discuss, and this shows up in people feigning headaches rather than saying they have their period; period products being hidden up sleeves; and supermarkets labeling period products as "sanitary items" and "feminine-hygiene products," implying that periods are dirty—they are not! Language matters, and this cements the idea in the subconscious that periods should be kept secret.

It can be hard to break free of the shame of periods, especially if it's been introduced from a young age—this is why shame-free menstrual education for all genders, from a young age, is important. If we have more understanding of how our bodies work, we'll be able to recognize what is normal and what our periods could be telling us.

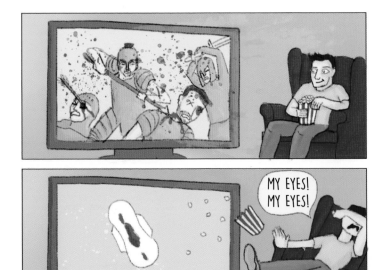

THE MENSTRUAL CYCLE

So what's going on? To understand what normal is,
it's important to understand what's happening.

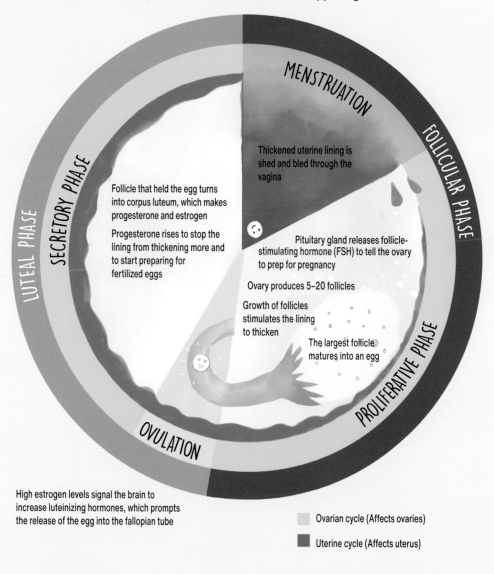

MENSTRUATION

FOLLICULAR PHASE

SECRETORY PHASE

LUTEAL PHASE

PROLIFERATIVE PHASE

OVULATION

Thickened uterine lining is
shed and bled through the
vagina

Follicle that held the egg turns
into corpus luteum, which makes
progesterone and estrogen

Progesterone rises to stop the
lining from thickening more and
to start preparing for
fertilized eggs

Pituitary gland releases follicle-
stimulating hormone (FSH) to tell the ovary
to prep for pregnancy

Ovary produces 5–20 follicles

Growth of follicles
stimulates the lining
to thicken

The largest follicle
matures into an egg

High estrogen levels signal the brain to
increase luteinizing hormones, which prompts
the release of the egg into the fallopian tube

Ovarian cycle (Affects ovaries)

Uterine cycle (Affects uterus)

CYCLE AWARENESS
(THINKING OF YOUR MENSTRUAL CYCLE AS SEASONS)

Each season represents a different part of the menstrual cycle. Everyone's cycle is different, but this thinking can help make sense of any cyclical mood by understanding what your hormones are doing. This can help you roughly plan for how you may be feeling at certain times of your cycle: you can warn loved ones to stay away, if you know you always get cranky at a certain time; or plan social events if you have a lot of energy at another time. Think of this as an example, not a hard-and-fast rule for everyone, and work out your own cyclical trends by monitoring how you feel each day.

KEY HORMONES
plummeting estrogen, progesterone levels rise but then drop drastically

FEATURES
feeling critical, sensitive; PMS, mood swings; energy decreasing as hormones drop; inner critic may be loudest here

WATCH OUT FOR
people who irritate you: you may find them extra irritating

KEY HORMONES
estrogen + testosterone peak

FEATURES
horny mode on, all eyes on me; feeling productive, energetic, magnetic; time for collaborating, working through difficult conversations

WATCH OUT FOR
saying yes to absolutely everything because you feel like you have the energy!

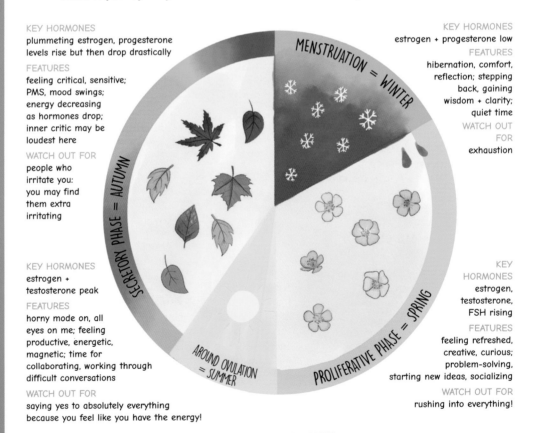

MENSTRUATION = WINTER

SECRETORY PHASE = AUTUMN

AROUND OVULATION = SUMMER

PROLIFERATIVE PHASE = SPRING

KEY HORMONES
estrogen + progesterone low

FEATURES
hibernation, comfort, reflection; stepping back, gaining wisdom + clarity; quiet time

WATCH OUT FOR
exhaustion

KEY HORMONES
estrogen, testosterone, FSH rising

FEATURES
feeling refreshed, creative, curious; problem-solving, starting new ideas, socializing

WATCH OUT FOR
rushing into everything!

THE HORMONES

Different hormones have different effects!

ESTROGEN

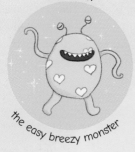

the easy breezy monster

- Boosts mood, confidence, and horniness levels
- Gives you energy to go go go!
- Makes you gloss over little annoyances
- Increases blood flow to the genitals + keeps vagina lubricated
- May give you healthy glowing skin due to association with increased collagen production, skin hydration, wound healing, and improved barrier function

PROGESTERONE

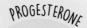

- Progesterone's role is to support pregnancy
- Can be calming
- Is a mild sedative + influences the sleep–wake cycle
- Plays a role in mood regulation

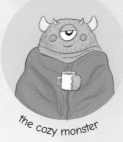

the cozy monster

TESTOSTERONE

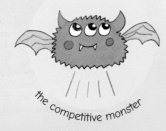

the competitive monster

- Increases libido
- Plays a role in metabolism + production of red blood cells, which give energy
- Preserves muscle mass
- Increases drive + motivation

IS THERE A NORMAL AGE TO START YOUR PERIOD?

Periods usually start around twelve, but some people can start as early as eight and others as late as eighteen.

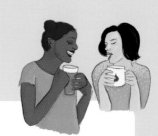

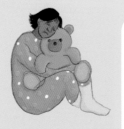

WHAT DOES NORMAL LOOK LIKE?

There is no one normal period, as periods can look different for everyone (genes and lifestyle play a big part), but to give you an idea, cycle lengths should be between twenty-four and thirty-five days. Longer cycles can be an indicator that ovulation is not occurring regularly. Shorter cycles can also indicate that ovulation is not occurring or that the ovaries contain fewer eggs. Bleeding typically lasts between three and seven days.

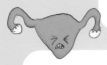

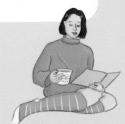

IS IT NORMAL TO FEEL PAIN?

While we all have a different tolerance to pain, please do get pain checked out, because it takes a global average of 7–9 years to be diagnosed with endometriosis. As I learned from the journalist Monica Karpinski, "Endometriosis presents with two sorts of symptoms: painful periods and/or pain during sex."

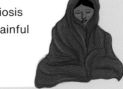

HOW MUCH BLOOD DO YOU LOSE ON YOUR PERIOD?

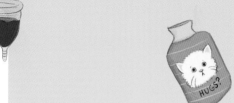

Between 5 ml and 80 ml. More than 80 ml is considered heavy bleeding.

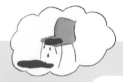

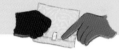

WHAT IS SPOTTING AND IS IT BAD?

Spotting is when there is blood outside of your period. Some spotting is normal, such as premenstrual spotting, which could be oxidized blood from a previous cycle for a couple of days; or ovulatory spotting (light-red/pink blood) for a couple of days. Spotting for longer than that may indicate more serious conditions, such as endometriosis, uterine fibroids, hypothyroidism, or cervical inflammation (which can be caused by infections). This should be investigated by a medical professional.

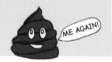

ME AGAIN!

THE PERIOD POOS!

If you find yourself needing to poo more around your period, that's normal. High levels of prostaglandins help to kick-start contractions to begin shedding the uterine lining, but they may also cause the intestinal muscles to contract, making you need to use the bathroom more often.

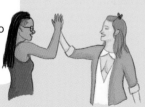

WHAT CAN YOUR PERIOD COLOR TELL YOU?

Light pink, red, dark red, and brown are all natural colors for periods.
However, different colors may also be indicators of other things!

ORANGE BLOOD
when mixed with cervical fluid,
blood can appear orange; this
could also be a sign of infection

DARK-RED BLOOD
may indicate the
end of the period
or that the blood
has been in the
uterus for a while

PINK BLOOD
can occur as your period begins
or ends; may sometimes indicate
low estrogen

BLACK/BROWN BLOOD
usually a sign of old blood
that has oxidized

GRAY BLOOD
could be related to an infection such
as bacterial vaginosis

SHOULD I TRACK MY PERIOD?

Period/cycle tracking provides a wealth of interesting information and can help you understand your body and its patterns. You can work out if you have a repetitive cycle length, which may help you predict which days you will start your period and may need to bring period products to work or school. You may become aware of certain days when you're a little more grumpy than usual, and can then prepare loved ones to stay away for a day. Tracking can help you work out sooner if you've missed a period. It can also be used as a form of birth control.

On the other hand, cycle tracking can help you understand your most fertile days and assist greatly in working out which days are best to conceive. Another pro to this practice is that you get to know what is normal for you and, if there's anything strange, you may notice it earlier and can then seek advice from a doctor or gynecologist.

They say that "knowledge is power," and to have a greater understanding of your own body is empowering, especially when you may need to communicate to a doctor when something is wrong, and particularly if said doctor dismisses your concerns—they are professionals and can give you their opinion, but they are not experiencing what is going on in your body.

HOW TO TRACK YOUR PERIOD

You can use a period tracking app,* a piece of paper, a spreadsheet, or whatever method you like and then choose what aspects you wish to monitor.

You could start by coloring in the days you bleed, tracking the length of your period, noting how heavy each bleed is, and whether there is any spotting. You could take this further and note your mood each day, how well you slept, if you experienced cramps/irritability/acne. Another step could be to take your basal body temperature, which could help work out your fertile days (however, this is not a 100 percent accurate fertility method). Or you could monitor your cervical fluid.

This information may come in handy one day and, if anything, it gives you that little bit more understanding of your body and what it's up to, so that you feel better prepared and more in control, rather than your body being in control of you.

* Be sure to look into the Ts and Cs and check which apps may be storing/sharing your data.

WHAT DOES THIS PAIN MEAN?

One reason people turn to Google is to research a particular symptom or a specific pain. So I interviewed Monica Karpinski, a journalist and the founder of The Femedic (a health media platform with reliable information for "women and people with vaginas"), to get those answers you're looking for. Or, rather, some tips on how to find the answers you're looking for amid all the misinformation online.

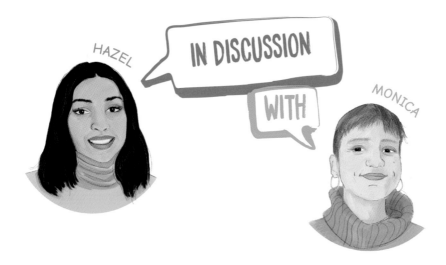

HAZEL

IN DISCUSSION WITH

MONICA

A lot of people google their pains and symptoms, but which sources of online information can you trust?

The most trustworthy organizations are the bigger medical institutions and the ones that publish clinical guidance—so the the National Institutes of Health (NIH), the Mayo Clinic, the Center for Diseases Control and Prevention (CDC), and the American College of Obstetricians and Gynecologists (ACOG). They collect all the evidence on a topic and rate its quality, finding out what's trustworthy, and then produce recommendations based on that. If you're looking at other websites, see what they're referencing and decide whether this is a source you want to trust:

• Are they getting that information from clinical guidance?
• Does it come from a medical study? Is it from a survey they carried out?
• Is it someone's personal experience? Everyone is an expert in their own experience.

A lot of mainstream health publishing misrepresents how much of an impact one factor has on one outcome. Correlation does not equal causation. For example (and I'm making this up), a study could show that among people who had heart attacks, more of them drank soft drinks, but that doesn't prove that soft drinks cause heart attacks. A newspaper could see that and suggest that "Soft drinks cause heart attacks," which completely misrepresents the situation.

How can you communicate and express your pain to a doctor or healthcare professional—especially with pain being subjective, and people having different pain thresholds?

Be as clear and specific as possible. What does the pain feel like?

- Is it dull?
- Is it throbbing?
- Is it burning?
- Does it come in waves?
- Is it there all the time?
- Is it triggered by something?

People will say, "Describe your pain on a scale of one to ten." That scale looks different for everybody and I think it has its drawbacks, but if you explain what a five means to you, then it can be useful. For example, I could say to a doctor, "I've got this pain in my pelvic area, and it's on pretty much all the time and it's a solid seven. And a five, for me, is like a headache that I can cope with if I take a painkiller." That kind of helps the doctor understand that it's above my threshold for normal coping, and therefore there might need to be some intervention. It's about letting them know exactly what's happening, so that it can help them come to a conclusion faster.

What do you think are some of the biases around the perception of who experiences pain?

The biases have been shaped by centuries of medical sexism and medical racism. The first female doctor in the US got her degree only in the 1840s, and the medical model for a long time was a white cisgender man. There was race science, which argued that people of color were biologically inferior because their physiology was different. And this was considered to be scientific at that time.

The institution of medicine is shaped by culture and society—it's not free from those biases. It's been built by white cisgender men, so that also introduces a bias against women. For example, "hysteria" in the eighteenth and nineteenth centuries was a diagnosis that doctors would give for women who weren't "behaving" in ways they felt women should behave. There are loads of quotes from doctors of that era—"She's not docile enough," "She's being too emotional," "She's being unruly"—because they expected women not to be those things. We still have the hangover from that today.

There are loads of statistics about pain not being taken seriously for that reason—because we're too emotional.

WOMEN

MORE LIKELY TO HAVE

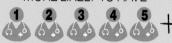 **+**

APPOINTMENTS
BEFORE DIAGNOSIS

CISGENDER WOMEN
50 PERCENT
HIGHER CHANCE
OF INCORRECT
INITIAL DIAGNOSIS
AFTER A HEART
ATTACK

LONGER
WAITING
TIMES IN
**EMERGENCY
ROOM**
FOR WOMEN

WOMEN
MORE LIKELY
THAN MEN
TO DIE IN
HOSPITAL OF

CONDITION

**PHYSICAL
MANIFESTATIONS
CAN BE DIFFERENT SO
ARE OFTEN MISSED**

NAUSEA   **BACK
PAIN**   **SHORTNESS
OF BREATH**

= MORE COMMON SYMPTOMS IN
WOMEN HAVING A HEART ATTACK*

30 TO 50 PERCENT

of women diagnosed
with depression
were misdiagnosed

29 percent

LESS LIKELY
than white patients
to be treated
WITH OPIOIDS

**BLACK
PATIENT**

22 percent

LESS LIKELY
than white patients to
get pain medication

So while culture is changing, studies are changing,
and awareness is changing, it will take a while for
that to come become normal. ■

However, people of all genders "can" experience the same or similar symptoms. Chest pain is still the most common.

HOW DO I PREPARE
FOR A CERVICAL SCREENING?

Having a cervical screening is an important part of your self-care. It checks the health of your cervix and helps to prevent cervical cancer. Different countries will ask you to go for a test at different ages. The American College of Obstetricians and Gynecologists recommends that women ages 21 to 65 get screened, also called a Pap test, every three to five years. (If you are male but have a cervix, you should still make an appoinment.) Cervical screening is not a test for cancer!

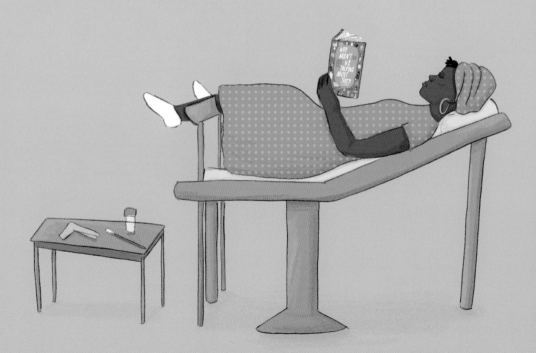

1 WHAT ARE THEY CHECKING FOR?

The cervical sample taken is checked for high-risk types of human papillomavirus (HPV), which can cause changes to the cells of your cervix. If HPV is not found, there won't be any further tests. If it is found, the sample is then checked to see if there have been any changes to your cells.

2 HOW TO PREPARE FOR THE APPOINTMENT

· Blood may interfere with the sample, so try to plan the appointment to avoid your period if possible.
· You don't need to shave! Medical professionals see loads of vulvas every day. Do whatever you feel comfortable with.
· Wear a skirt, a dress, some sweatpants, or something that can be taken off with ease or lifted up—maybe not a playsuit with laces, zips, and forty-eight buttons.

3 WHAT TO EXPECT AT THE APPOINTMENT

· Your nurse or sample-taker should explain a bit about the test and give you the opportunity to ask any questions.
· They will give you some privacy to undress from the waist down, if you need to, and provide a sheet if you wish to cover yourself.
· You will be asked to lie down, on your back or side.
· Once you feel ready, they will start the test by inserting a speculum (the medical instrument used to dilate you) into your vagina so that they can see the cervix.
· A small, soft brush will be inserted and they will gently rotate it to take a sample.
· The brush is then removed and put into a sample tube.

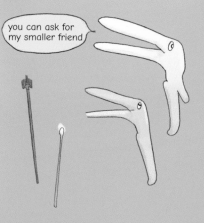

you can ask for my smaller friend

4 THE RESULTS

It will take two to six weeks to get your results.

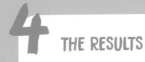
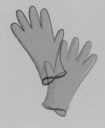

5 WHAT HAPPENS NEXT: WILL I BE ASKED TO COME BACK, AND SHOULD I BE WORRIED?

The test is for high-risk HPV cells and cervical cell changes. There are a few potential results:

HPV found, with cell changes

you have high-risk HPV and cell changes, so you will be asked to go for a colposcopy test to check what is going on.

No HPV found

you don't have high-risk HPV, so you'll be invited back in three or five years' time for another check-up.

HPV found, but no cell changes

you have high-risk HPV, but no cervical cell changes, so you will be asked back for a cervical screening sooner, often after a year, to keep an eye on things.

SMEAR FEAR

According to a study of 2,000 women by Jo's Cervical Cancer Trust, one of the most common reasons women missed their appointments was due to body shame and embarrassment. Sample-takers see many vulvas and vaginas—they're there to help, not to judge!

Some people worry about the test due to a fear of penetration or sexual trauma, or have conditions that make penetration painful or impossible. If someone tells you they have missed a test, talk to them from a place of empathy rather than judgment. The discourse around cervical screening can be very judgmental.

If pain is something you are concerned about, there are several things you can do to make you feel more at ease:

 Have an initial consultation appointment, so that you feel more comfortable with the sample-taker.

 See if there's an option to take the speculum home, or get a speculum to practice inserting it.

 Book a double appointment, so that you can have more time to prepare and ask any questions.

 Ask for a smaller speculum if you're worried about pain.

 Discuss painkillers or anesthetic creams.

 Discuss vaginal moisturizers if you have painful conditions such as lichen sclerosus.

 Bring along someone you feel comfortable with.

 Use techniques to distract you—hypnosis, a podcast, or music.

 Remember that you can say no at any time: you are in control.

 Plan a treat for yourself after the appointment, so that you have something to look forward to.

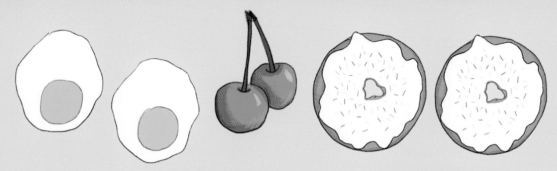

HOW CAN I CHECK MY BOOBS OR BALLS?

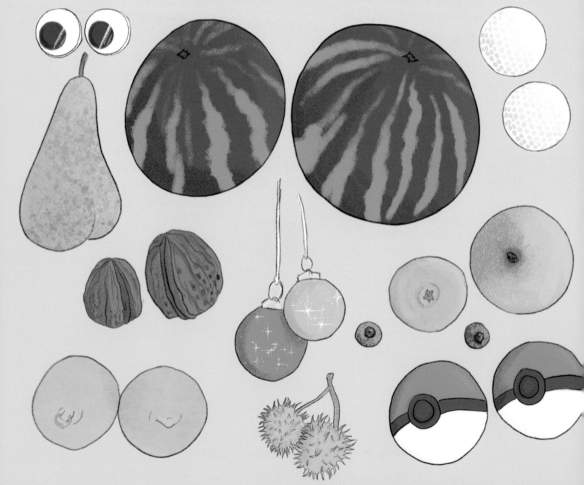

One in eight women will be diagnosed with breast cancer throughout their lifetime in the US. However, one in 100 breast cancer cases occur in men, so it does affect all genders. (Currently there is very little research into how the stats look for transgender people.)

PROSTATE CANCER

Prostate cancer affects one in eight men in the US. Unfortunately, it doesn't really have any visible symptoms, but if you're over fifty, Black or mixed Black ethnicity, or have a family history of cancer, you are more likely to get it.

Certain symptoms sometimes show up, including an increase in the amount you need to urinate, the urgency with which you need to urinate, needing to urinate at night, difficulty in starting to urinate, and a decreased force in urination. However, these can also be caused by other factors such as aging or an enlarged prostate. And many times prostate cancer is symptomless. That's why if you're in the higher-risk categories it is good to get frequent checks. And if you're concerned, do get it checked out.

TESTICULAR CANCER

While much rarer, you can check for testicular cancer yourself (see page 162).

BREAST CANCER

Get to know your own normal, which is different for everyone. Your chest changes through puberty, pregnancy, breastfeeding, and menopause, due to different levels of hormones. Feel and look around your breast tissue, armpits, and collarbones to find any noticeable changes. If you need some help, get someone you'd feel comfortable with checking your breasts/chest for you, and communicate what feels okay.

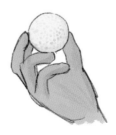
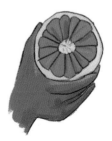

BOOBS

NIPPLE DISCHARGE

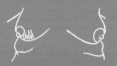

CHANGES IN SKIN TEXTURE
(PUCKERING/DIMPLING)

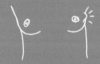

LUMPS AND THICKENING

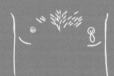

NIPPLE INVERSION OR
CHANGES IN DIRECTION

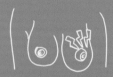

CONSTANT UNUSUAL
PAIN IN THE BREAST OR
ARMPIT

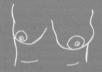

A SUDDEN CHANGE IN
SIZE OR SHAPE

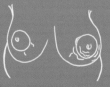

BLEEDING NIPPLES

If anything feels out
of the ordinary, book an
appointment with your doctor,
so that they can give you
reassurance or check for
cancerous tissue.

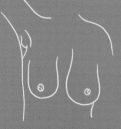

SWELLING IN THE
ARMPIT/COLLARBONE

A RASH OR CRUSTING
OF THE NIPPLE OR
SURROUNDING AREA

BALLS

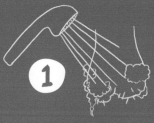

GET YOUR BALLS WARM—A HOT SHOWER IS RECOMMENDED.

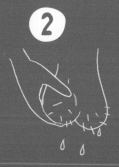

Check monthly. If anything feels out of the ordinary, book an appointment with your doctor, so that they can give you reassurance or check for cancerous tissue.

ROLL ONE TESTICLE BETWEEN YOUR THUMB AND FINGER TO CHECK FOR:

OR SWELLING

LUMPS

PAIN

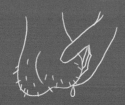

REPEAT WITH TESTICLE TWO.

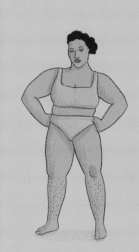
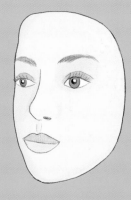
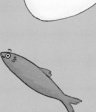
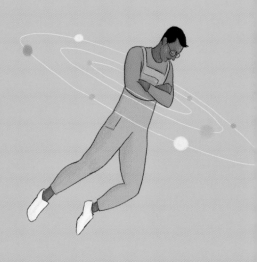
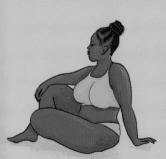

the self +

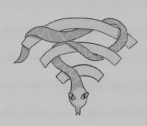
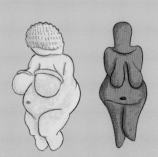
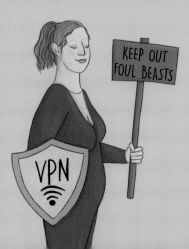

KEEP OUT
FOUL BEASTS

VPN

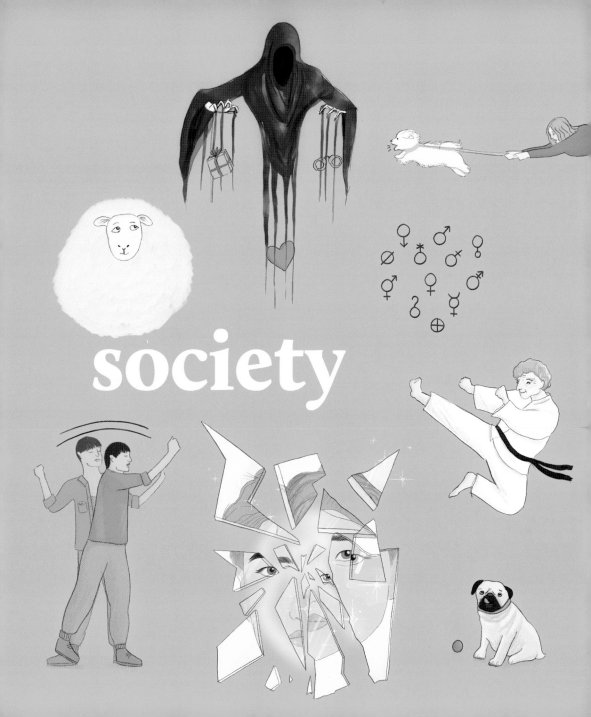

society

We don't get to decide where we're born or who we're born as. It's a total lottery. The society we're born into comes with a conditioned set of rules around how you're supposed to behave and who you're supposed to be, who matters and who doesn't. And you may feel like you fit in quite well and have many advantages in life or you may feel like you're not able to be yourself.

This section aims to question which aspects of society's teachings may not be working for you, figuring out how you can find peace with yourself, as well as a reminder to offer others the same empathy you'd like to receive and understand you also have your own biases and may not always be right. I'm tackling some concerns that have always been around: identity, ego, security, body image; but in the digital age these have perhaps become more apparent.

I also want to equip you with some necessary knowledge to protect you from people in society who may want to cause you harm. We live in an age when everything seems so divided—perhaps, as the human race, we've always been that way—yet we need each other more than ever.

THOSE BRIEF CONNECTIONS WITH PEOPLE YOU MAY NEVER SEE AGAIN

The person you once chatted with for the whole bus ride home

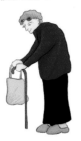

The really great yoga teacher

The dog from the park

Your sibling's ex

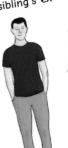

The nice nurse who gave you candy for being brave

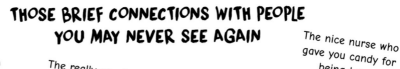

The person you stood behind in a line

Your ex's mom

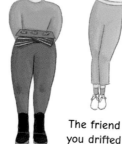

The barista you used to chat with every day

The girl whose eye you caught on the train

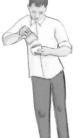

The baby that cried on the flight

The friend you drifted away from

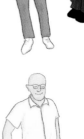

The person who you flirted with and crushed on—but it was never meant to be

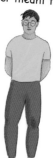

The school crossing guard

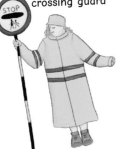

The homeless man who sat outside the supermarket

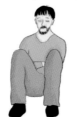

The work friends who made work great

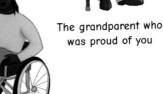

The grandparent who was proud of you

The vacation cat you adopted for a week

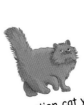

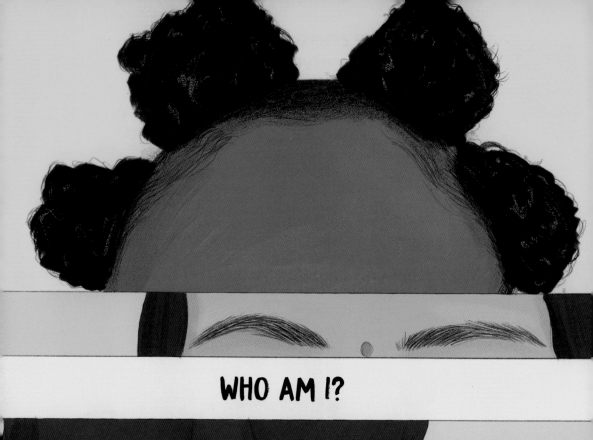
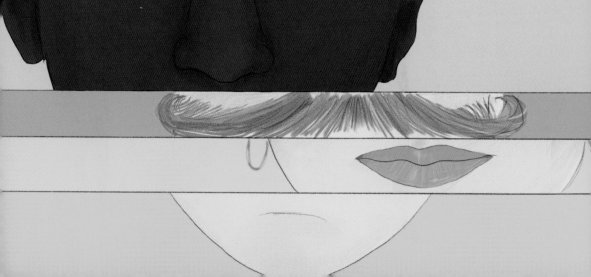

When someone asks you to describe yourself, the chances are that you align yourself to a group that people understand, a social identity—possibly one of the big eight socially constructed identities (see below) or whatever characteristic you most relate to.

We could go into deep philosophical discussions about what truly makes you *you*—if you lost your leg, would you still be you? Yes. If you lost your memory, would you still be you? Possibly. Who we really are is a culmination of how we dress, speak, and express ourselves; the groups that we align ourselves with; our experiences; who we believe we are; and our continuous sense of character. Identity is more pronounced when we compare ourselves to others—for instance, what separates me from that person? We find comfort in groups that are similar to us and cling closely to them.

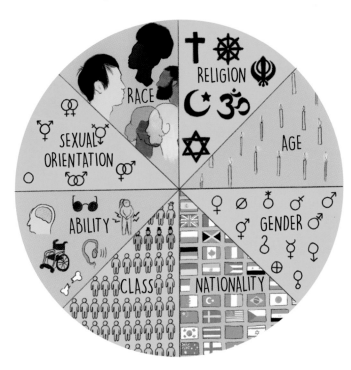

IDENTITY CRISIS

Perhaps an identity crisis actually reveals more about who we think we are—when something you strongly identified with is changed or taken away, you're forced to re-examine who you are.

An identity crisis happens in the face of change. A new job, or loss of a job, can drive you towards the person you want to be, or further away from who you believed you were. Divorce may make people question who they are outside of a relationship. New parents can feel a loss of self, when their new identity revolves solely around being Mom or Dad.

However, the opposite is also true: a change can bring a sense of self, fulfilling a part of you that you thought was missing. Every change shifts our identity, as it makes us re-examine ourselves. A midlife or quarter-life crisis can occur due to a shift that makes you feel unhappy about your age, fear the inevitability of death, or feel like you haven't accomplished enough.

SIGNS OF AN IDENTITY CRISIS

- Feeling dissatisfaction
- Struggling to find purpose
- Questioning your character
- Unable to find passion

HOW TO RE-FIND/RE-CREATE YOURSELF

Imagine the ideal you in a parallel universe where there were no external expectations, only guaranteed success. Get a piece of paper and don't hold back with this exercise! Be as detailed as possible. This is for your eyes only.

Step 1: Write out: Who are they? What are they doing? Where are they living? What is a day in the life for them?

Step 2: Write out how the two of you are different.
Is it money related? Is it career related? Is it health related?
Are the people around you different? Are the two of you in different locations?

Step 3: Write out how you can bridge the gap between you.
- Should you be doing anything differently to what you're doing now?
- Change is uncomfortable; if applicable, in what way is your comfort zone holding you back?
- Do you have an inner saboteur that fears failure or succeeding?
- Do the people that you surround yourself with lift you up or drag you down?
- Are there any clear first steps to help you embark on this journey, or is there something you can work towards?

While plans often go wrong or awry, it can be helpful to have a direction to guide you, that you can revisit. And remember, throughout your life you're allowed to change your mind and that's completely normal and natural.

EXISTING IN THE IN-BETWEEN

It can be hard to exist in that liminal space between two boxes. People who identify as mixed race, for example, may feel shunned by both communities—not enough of one or the other to be allowed into either group. It's complex, because even within the community of people with dual heritage, everyone's experience is different—and I think that's the key. On the one hand, of course you're allowed to be proud of both parts! On the other hand, colorism and judgments around you from those with racist beliefs do occur in everyday life—and the area in which you find yourself living can have a large impact on how you're perceived and even on your self-perception.

Mixed-race people have different skin colors—some dark, some light-skinned, some white-passing—which have an impact on day-to-day interactions, based on people's assumptions and stereotypes concerning how you look. Some mixed-race people with a more "ambiguous" look may experience rejection and discrimination from both sides of their heritage, while others have one part of their heritage completely ignored, due to having more pronounced features from one side or the other. And everyone has a different experience of that.

Illustration based on the gray dot optical illusion and my personal experience of my skin color against the backdrop of the all-white village I grew up in vs. the multicultural city I find myself in now. It's all relative.

NON-BINARY GENDER IDENTITY

Non-binary people who don't neatly fit into the gender binary of man or woman also face discrimination, with people trying to confine them to a box of either/or.

The Voice Online asked Dr. Ronx Ikharia, a queer, non-binary, trans emergency medicine doctor, for advice to give young people about managing their identities, and Dr. Ronx replied with this invaluable advice: "One of the things I say to young people is take your time—and that goes for everything. For example, I changed my pronouns to 'they/them' earlier on this year. I recognize that it's going to take time for elders or the other people in my life to adopt that, so I'm patient. In terms of visibility, I always say to people that you don't owe anybody anything, you owe yourself everything."

In a separate interview with *Attitude* magazine, Dr. Ronx disclosed how it felt hearing the phrase "You don't look like a doctor" from a young Black boy who had genuinely never seen a Black doctor before. They said, "It birthed my desire to take those kinds of features and intersections of myself and use them as a positive, leaning into being a role model for those who perhaps hadn't seen a queer, Black, androgynous, LGBTQI doctor being allowed to exist alongside everyone else as a professional, and be visible as a TV personality."

While non-binary and transgender people have always existed, it feels like only recently there's been a shift in thinking about language and more inclusion. See the following page for some terminology to familiarize yourself with.

GENDER TERMINOLOGY

SEX
biological status based on anatomy
(male, female, intersex)

GENDER
social construct of typical roles and behaviors
(male, female, non-binary)

GENDER IDENTITY
one's own internal sense of gender
(male, female, no gender, non-binary)

GENDER EXPRESSION
how someone portrays gender outwardly
(masculine, feminine, androgynous/other)

CISGENDER
someone whose gender identity aligns
with the sex assigned at birth

TRANSGENDER
someone whose gender identity differs
from the sex assigned at birth

AGENDER
someone who does not identify
with any gender

NON-BINARY/GENDERQUEER
someone whose gender identity doesn't fit into
the categories of man and woman

GENDERFLUID
someone whose gender identity varies over time

GENDER DYSPHORIA
feelings ranging from unease to distress,
resulting from incongruence between one's sex
assigned at birth and one's gender identity

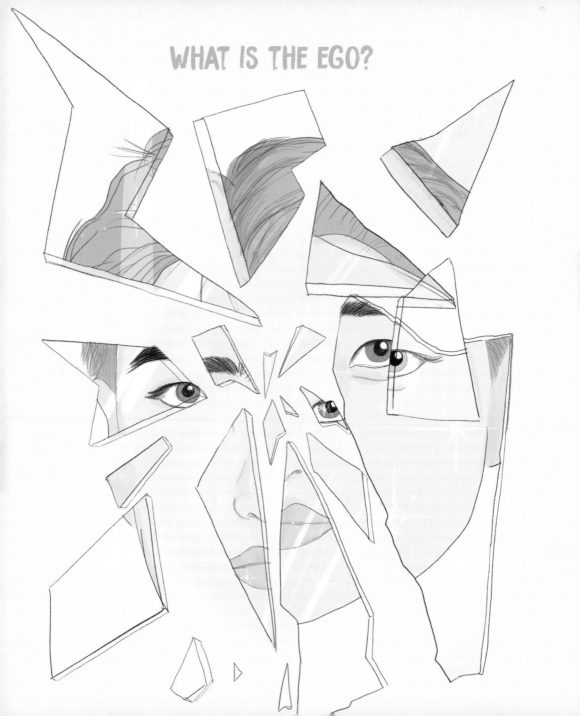

WHAT IS THE EGO?

Ego is the Latin word for "I" and, simply put, the ego refers to our sense of self. It acts like a filter on the world around us, and is often imbued with our own sense of self-importance and the narratives we create about ourselves and society.

As children, we think the world is all about us. As we get older, we realize it's not, but the ego can keep us in a state of self-importance. We are all the main characters in our own stories.

WHEN THE EGO IS DESTRUCTIVE

The destructive part happens when we are controlled by our ego: maybe you feel superior to others, or maybe it makes you play the victim. It can leave us struggling with our identity. It can take our concern with self-image and turn it into obsession.

Perhaps that's what you commonly think of when you hear the word "ego." It's feeling like you have a sexy body. It's being smug about having a nice car. It's showing off your awards, achievements, and accolades. It's an inflated sense of self through your social media follower count. It's anything that feeds your ego to the point where you feel superior. While it's perfectly fine to enjoy those things and to appreciate that you have attributes you're proud of or that bring you joy, when they leave you with a feeling of superiority or become part of your identity, that's the ego rearing its head.

The contrast occurs when someone doesn't feel good in themselves or feels inferior—it's the opposite end of the spectrum, but has a similar result of comparison to others. If you feel threatened by someone else's success, bitter about someone's appearance, or envious of their possessions, that's the ego popping up again, which wants you to feel more important, better, more acknowledged.

The other add-on to this is judging someone else's materialism, which is a more subtle moral superiority: "I'm better than this person because I'm not concerned with material things"; "I'm more eco-conscious . . . I'm more moral . . . I'm more self-aware . . . I'm more loving." This still results in a feeling of superiority, judging yourself as better in relation to other people.

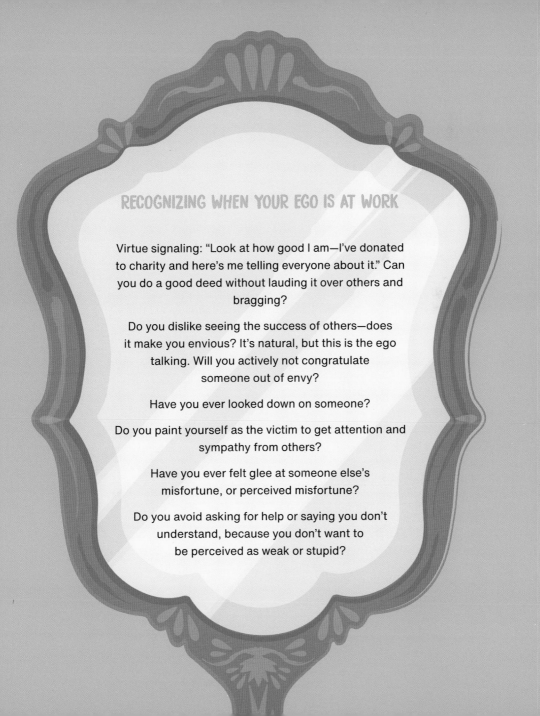

RECOGNIZING WHEN YOUR EGO IS AT WORK

Virtue signaling: "Look at how good I am—I've donated to charity and here's me telling everyone about it." Can you do a good deed without lauding it over others and bragging?

Do you dislike seeing the success of others—does it make you envious? It's natural, but this is the ego talking. Will you actively not congratulate someone out of envy?

Have you ever looked down on someone?

Do you paint yourself as the victim to get attention and sympathy from others?

Have you ever felt glee at someone else's misfortune, or perceived misfortune?

Do you avoid asking for help or saying you don't understand, because you don't want to be perceived as weak or stupid?

OUR EGO IS UNWILLING TO CHANGE

Ego is also rooted in a very rigid idea that we have about ourselves and the world—in a debate, people generally arrive not with the idea that their minds will be changed, but that they'll be able to articulate their own views more eloquently and will ultimately have them judged as more correct than the other side's.

In our lives we are the main characters, with others as side characters, even villains—in fact, it is quite rare to accept responsibility when we have approached a situation in the wrong light. We may be the villain of someone else's story, and that's a tough pill to swallow. When feeling alone, it can be natural to start projecting outwards, thinking, "Why have none of my friends reached out to me? Can't they sense I'm alone?" Yet they have their own lives and their own concerns and they may also be feeling the same way.

IS THE EGO ALWAYS NEGATIVE?

We've evolved to develop ego as it keeps us safe by being concerned with the self, thus giving us the will to survive and the desire to succeed. We don't want to get rid of it. But we can have a healthier relationship with it and not be all-consumed by a fragile sense of self.

A healthy ego can give you confidence and self-belief as opposed to a big, dominating ego that displays arrogance and boastfulness. You will be more open to constructive criticism, too, as it's less likely to dent your pride.

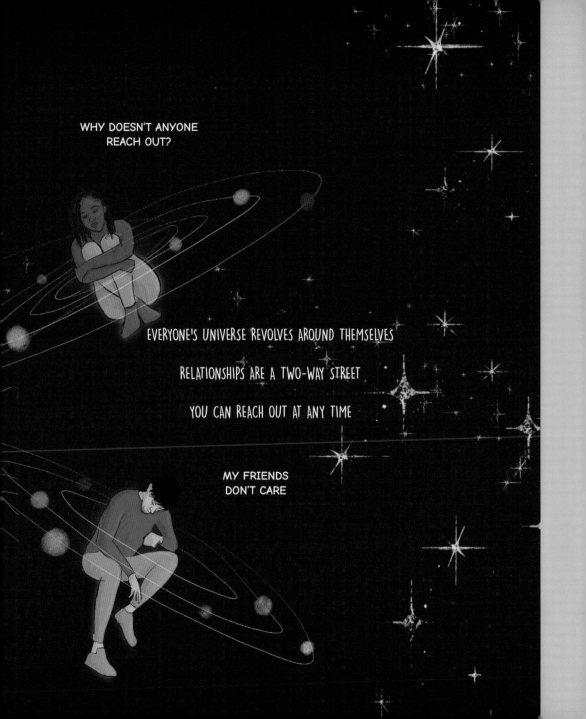

WHAT CAN WE DO TO KEEP OUR EGOS IN CHECK?

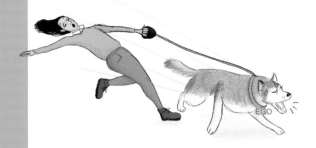

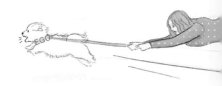

We can surround ourselves with others: people who know more than us, to remind us that we can still grow, learn more, and that we don't know everything. We are not the best! And we sometimes need a dose of humility.

We can listen more to others and get a wider perspective on the world. Do you leave a conversation thinking the other person didn't say anything? Perhaps you spoke a great deal about yourself, without leaving room for anyone else or even inquiring about the other person. With other viewpoints come opportunities to reflect on how yours is not the one true way, and this leads to opportunities for empathy.

We can remind ourselves that we're not that important, we're a small speck in the vast universe, and we're not here for that long—we're here and we die, and we won't be remembered in a couple of hundred years. Perhaps that sounds incredibly bleak, but I think it's also liberating. The Australian nurse Bronnie Ware asked people on their deathbeds what their biggest regret was. She found many similar themes: around working too hard, not having the courage to live their true selves or to express their feelings. A lot of that comes from ego and worrying what others think.

WHAT IS NEURODIVERGENCE?

Not all of us experience the various processes that I describe in this book in the same way. "Neurodiversity" refers to differences in cognitive style and the idea that diversity in brains is common among humans. The neurodiverse brain works differently from the neurotypical brain. Neurodiversity is a term that was first coined by Judy Singer, an autism activist, "to articulate the needs of people with autism who did not want to be defined by a disability label but wished to be seen instead as neurologically different."

This suggests that neurodiverse conditions are a part of who a person is and shouldn't be changed or cured. Rather, we should find ways to adapt to neurodiverse people and accept that they have different ways of learning and expression.

CONDITIONS COMMONLY RECOGNIZED UNDER THE "NEURODIVERSE" UMBRELLA

Autism
(or Autism Spectrum Disorder/ASD)
a broad range of conditions characterized by challenges with social skills, repetitive behaviors, speech, and/or non-verbal communication

Attention Deficit Hyperactivity Disorder (ADHD)
a condition characterized by trouble with concentration and focus, or impulsiveness

Tourette's syndrome and tic disorders
disorders characterized by sudden, repetitive, and unwanted movements or vocal sounds

Dyslexia
a learning disorder that involves difficulty in reading due to problems with interpreting letters and words

Dyspraxia
(developmental coordination disorder)
a condition that affects physical coordination and motor skills

Dyscalculia
a specific and persistent difficulty in understanding numbers

Dysgraphia
a specific learning disorder in written expression

Synesthesia
a condition whereby someone experiences things through their senses in an unusual way—for example, by hearing color or seeing music

SYNESTHESIA

DYSLEXIA

AUTISTIC TRAITS TO BE AWARE OF

Everyone's experience of autism is different, so not all of these traits are applicable to every autistic person.

- Finding **social communication with neurotypical people difficult**, because some autistic people struggle with non-verbal cues, with responding when spoken to, understanding micro-expressions, staying on topic in conversations, and decoding white lies or sarcasm. They may believe people's words rather than reading between the lines, and struggle with taking turns in conversations and using tone of voice (like different volumes for the playground and the classroom).
- Some autistic people find **emotions overwhelming**, as it may be difficult to connect feeling to an emotion.
- Some people are **hypersensitive** to different sensory stimuli and find certain sounds, textures, tastes, and sights—such as flashing lights, or being touched in one spot for a long time—overwhelming.
- Other people are **hyposensitive**: this is the other end of the spectrum, where there is difficulty in identifying sensations such as hunger and pain, and they may need to seek out more sensory input.

- **Stimming** is a common form of trying to rebalance sensory output, where some autistic people self-soothe in ways such as rocking.
- Some autistic people are very **proficient in certain areas, yet find other things extremely difficult**.
- Some people **struggle with executive function** and with working towards a goal, such as time management and flexibility.
- Others can be highly sensitive to change.

These traits are on a sliding scale—each autistic person may experience them to different degrees.

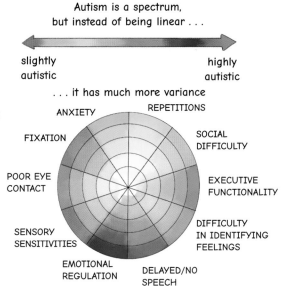

Autism is a spectrum, but instead of being linear . . .

slightly autistic   highly autistic

. . . it has much more variance

ANXIETY
REPETITIONS
FIXATION
SOCIAL DIFFICULTY
POOR EYE CONTACT
EXECUTIVE FUNCTIONALITY
DIFFICULTY IN IDENTIFYING FEELINGS
SENSORY SENSITIVITIES
EMOTIONAL REGULATION
DELAYED/NO SPEECH

ADHD TRAITS TO BE AWARE OF

Similarly, everyone's experience of ADHD is different, so not all traits will be applicable to each person.

- Inattentiveness, such as becoming easily distracted, appearing forgetful, and being unable to stick to tasks that are tedious or time-consuming
- Hyperactivity and impulsiveness, such as fidgeting and being unable to sit still, excessive physical movement, acting without thinking, interrupting conversations, and risk-taking
- Mood swings

ADHD AND AUTISM IN WOMEN + MASKING

Autism and ADHD are often recognized less in women than in men. That could be due to a couple of reasons. First, autism and ADHD symptoms have been less studied in girls and women, so the ways in which they present differently are not always picked up on. Tests used to diagnose autism and ADHD are still based on studies that were conducted on white autistic boys, which leads to lower diagnosis in girls. Second, even though it is the same disorder and affects the same brain regions in women and men, the symptoms can present differently, due to social differences.

According to Jessica McCabe, who hosts the YouTube channel How to ADHD, whereas many boys may develop problems such as rule-breaking and aggression, indications of girls having ADHD may be slightly more subtle; they "might take the form of racing thoughts, speaking before thinking, talking quickly." A lot of women and girls get misdiagnosed with depression and bipolar disorder and may be labelled as "spacey, messy, clumsy, weird, lazy, and irresponsible."

There may also be pressure to mask symptoms—a social survival strategy used by some neurodivergent people where they emulate behaviors that are deemed more socially acceptable in a neurotypical society—due to expectations to act in a certain way. This goes for many people with differences in brain function and is common in both ADHD and autism. People may mimic gestures, rehearse conversations, suppress certain behaviors, and force eye contact to be more like those of others.

If you're questioning whether you're autistic or have ADHD, or simply want to understand more, I highly recommend I Am Paying Attention, a community-driven platform set up by Jess Joy and

Charlotte Mia, which provides resources and self-assessment questionnaires on both autism and ADHD.

Another resource to look at is the website Embrace Autism, which provides further quality information about autism.

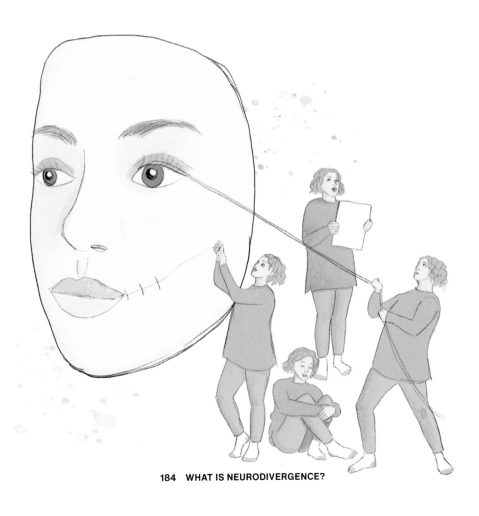

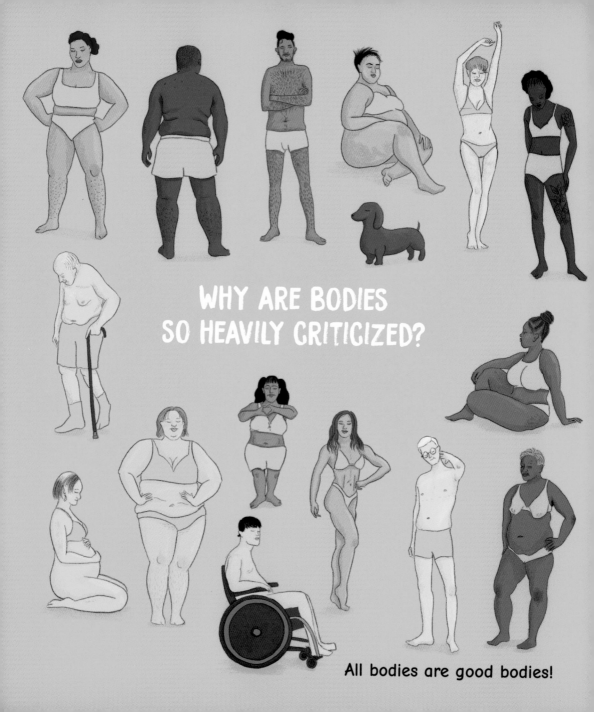

WHY ARE BODIES
SO HEAVILY CRITICIZED?

All bodies are good bodies!

CHASING PERFECTION

A Gallup poll reported that, as of November 2021, only 53 percent of Americans said that their weight was "about right," with 47 percent trying to change it.

Being bombarded by images of the "perfect body" can make us scrutinize how our own body measures up. Once an idea of perfect has been shaped, we start seeing imperfections everywhere, in others as well as ourselves. And it can start young—we pick up on which bodies are visible and which ones are demonized in films, media, and the way our family members talk about their own bodies.

For years, the scrutiny of famous women's bodies in magazines, with the cruel tradition of "before" and "after" photos splashed over front covers, has created a culture whereby women are not allowed to age, sag, show postpartum body weight, have cellulite, or be anything other than thin and young, for fear of ridicule. Perhaps people find comfort in the perceived flaws of others (especially in seemingly "flawless" celebrities) in order to feel better about themselves, but it's a harmful cycle, where you can internalize these messages. Check yourself when you're making yourself feel better by tearing others down.

FAT BODIES

A byproduct of the quest for the perfect body is the demonization of fat bodies. We've been told that being fat is awful. In film and TV, fat people are often used for laughs or are representative of evil, while romantic leads are, on the whole, thin. The discrimination against fat people has been justified in the name of being concerned for their health, but that same concern isn't applied to others, such as slimmer people who are living unhealthy lifestyles. It comes from a fatphobic place. With a flood of diet culture everywhere, no wonder fatphobia exists. From family members obsessing about their weight, to fad quick-fix diets and TV shows about people losing weight through extreme bootcamps, fatphobia surrounds us. Plus it has been proven that the discrimination itself is harmful to fat people's mental and physical health.

"Racism, sexism, ableism, homo- and transphobia, ageism, fatphobia are algorithms created by humans' struggle to make peace with the body."
SONYA RENEE TAYLOR—FOUNDER OF THE BODY IS NOT AN APOLOGY

The world caters to the thin: in clothing sizes, seat sizes, and dating preference. On the podcast *Should I Delete That?*, *Great British Baking Show* finalist Laura Adlington discussed how there is both a feeling of invisibility and hypervisibility: "I wish there was just more empathy for people in bigger bodies . . . You're invisible in that you don't matter—you're overlooked in healthcare, in jobs. But at the same time you're made aware of your bigness and how much of a problem it is."

POSTPARTUM BODIES

Creating life is magical. Throughout pregnancy there is a focus on giving care to whoever is pregnant, then straight afterwards all the attention is on the baby, even though the pregnant person's body has just gone through an ordeal and continues to, through breastfeeding (if they choose), moving organs back into place, healing from a C-section. Plus the pressure to lose the pregnancy weight and bounce back is unfairly rife. Take good care of people who've just had a baby. They deserve so much love and appreciation.

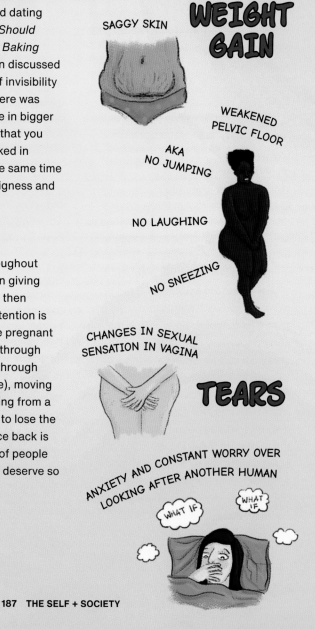

SAGGY SKIN

WEIGHT GAIN

WEAKENED PELVIC FLOOR

AKA NO JUMPING

NO LAUGHING

NO SNEEZING

CHANGES IN SEXUAL SENSATION IN VAGINA

TEARS

ANXIETY AND CONSTANT WORRY OVER LOOKING AFTER ANOTHER HUMAN

WHAT IF
WHAT IF
WHAT IF

WHAT WE'RE NOT TOLD ABOUT POSTPARTUM BODIES

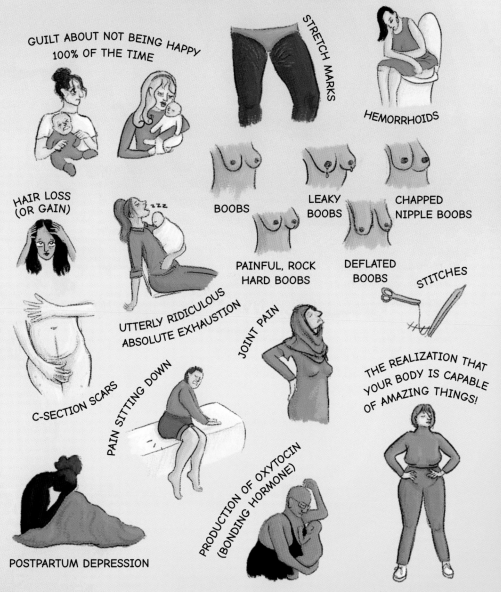

HOW CAN I BE MORE AT PEACE WITH MY BODY?

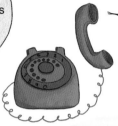

1. Focus on the things you do like about yourself.

2. Cut out the negative self-talk. Would you talk to a friend that way? Would a friend talk to you that way? So why be so harsh on yourself?

3. Do you ever look at photos of yourself from years gone by and think "Wow, I looked great," but remember that at the time you still felt not good enough? Imagine what "future you" would say to current you!

I WISH I WAS THINNER

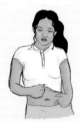

ARGH! A GRAY HAIR! A WRINKLE! I'M GETTING SO OLD.

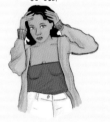

WHAT WAS I WORRIED ABOUT? I WISH I STILL LOOKED LIKE THAT!

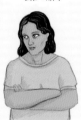

WHY DID I WASTE SO MUCH TIME WORRYING ABOUT HOW I LOOK?

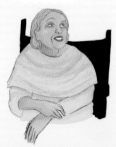

I FINALLY FEEL COMFORTABLE IN MY SKIN. I WISH I'D FOUND THIS CONFIDENCE EARLIER

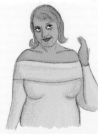

4. Remember, beauty and body standards have changed throughout history and across cultures. Your body is not a trend.

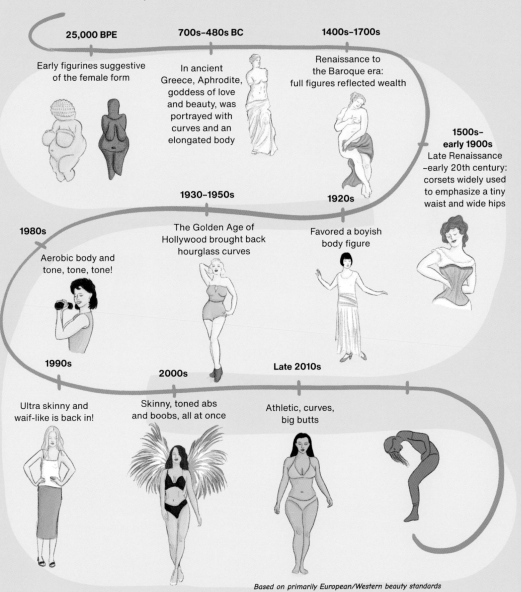

25,000 BPE

Early figurines suggestive of the female form

700s–480s BC

In ancient Greece, Aphrodite, goddess of love and beauty, was portrayed with curves and an elongated body

1400s–1700s

Renaissance to the Baroque era: full figures reflected wealth

1500s–early 1900s
Late Renaissance –early 20th century: corsets widely used to emphasize a tiny waist and wide hips

1930–1950s

The Golden Age of Hollywood brought back hourglass curves

1920s

Favored a boyish body figure

1980s

Aerobic body and tone, tone, tone!

1990s

Ultra skinny and waif-like is back in!

2000s

Skinny, toned abs and boobs, all at once

Late 2010s

Athletic, curves, big butts

Based on primarily European/Western beauty standards

5. Remember, people post their best photos on social media, not their worst!

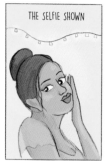

THE SELFIE SHOWN

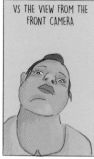

VS THE VIEW FROM THE FRONT CAMERA

6. Follow people on social media who promote body positivity and mute those who make you feel bad about yourself.

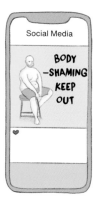

Social Media

BODY
—SHAMING
KEEP
OUT

7. Avoid the comparison game and taking part in the media's obsession over (specifically/especially) women's bodies.

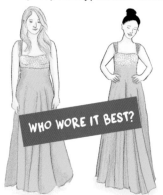

WHO WORE IT BEST?

(They both look great, leave them be.)

8. Buy clothes for the body you have, not the body you're trying to get. It's extra pressure to not like yourself in the present.

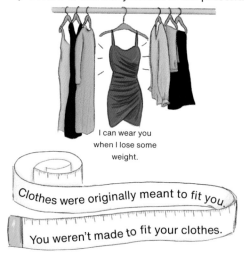

I can wear you when I lose some weight.

Clothes were originally meant to fit you.

You weren't made to fit your clothes.

9. Embrace body neutrality. When body positivity—loving your body—seems like too much pressure, body neutrality can be a great middle ground. Accept and appreciate your body for its function, not what it looks like.

YOUR BODY IS AMAZING!

When you receive information through one of your senses, the signal travels from your nerves to your brain at over 100 miles per hour

The average human eye can differentiate between roughly 1 million different colors

We glow! We emit light, we just can't see it

Your heart pumps 5.5 liters of blood per minute. So, during an average lifetime, it will pump nearly 1.5 million barrels of blood—enough to fill 200 train cars

We can grow life!

Melanin is a natural sunscreen!

Your skin can be grafted from one part of your body to grow on another part. It is the human body's largest organ and is constantly renewing itself

Your bones are stronger than steel

Our bodies are made from stardust!

The human body can adapt to its surrounding environment: for example, some people living in high altitudes have developed the ability to produce more red blood cells to help them absorb more oxygen

The odds of you existing are one in 400 quadrillion, at least. It is a miracle you exist!

HOW CAN I STAY SECURE ONLINE?

In a highly digital world, putting digital security and privacy in place is a must! There are people who want to exploit you, blackmail you, swindle you out of money, dox you, or use your information against you—for example to punish you for having an abortion, in places where abortions are illegal. I want to give you the tools and warning signs to help you spot scams and make it harder for people to hack you and exploit you.

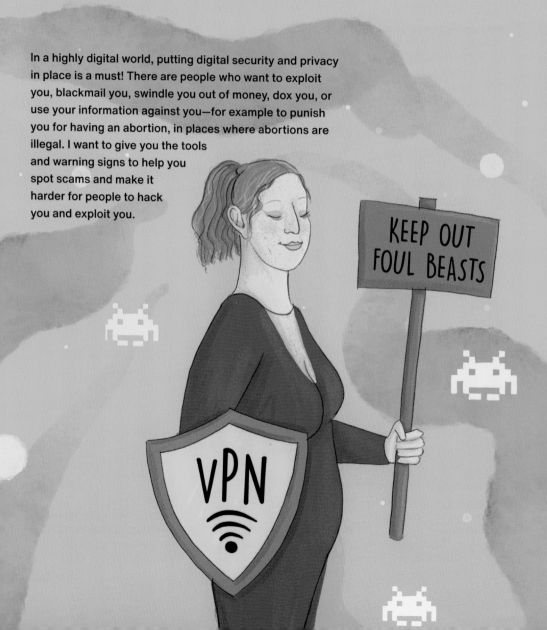

PRACTICAL DIGITAL SECURITY TIPS

To make it harder for others to get into your accounts and access your information:

 Don't open mail from strangers or click strange-looking links.

Do the updates: they can fix bugs and issues with operating systems.

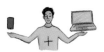 **Use strong passwords**, not pet names, birthdays or "password." Try a password generator or use three random words. Use different passwords for different services, so that if one is compromised, other services are secure. A password manager is recommended, so that you don't have to remember them all.

Turn on two-factor authentication: even if someone gets your password, they won't be able to get into that service.

Ideally, avoid unsecured wi-fi: anyone with a special app, such as Wireshark, can see what you're searching for if you're on an unencrypted website.

 Back up your data and files in case of an accident or virus. If you become a victim of malware, you might not get your data and files back.

Avoid online quizzes: some of these cleverly ask "random" questions that are actually gathering the answers to common security questions.

Educate your family: a virus can get into your network through your family devices and onto yours, if you're using the same router.

HOW TO CHECK
IF A WEBSITE
IS ENCRYPTED
on the search
bar, check for a
padlock or https, not
just http—the s is
important.

RECOGNIZING SCAM TACTICS

Scammers work by manipulating people through unethical social engineering. Scammers usually offer a reward, create a feeling of trust, or raise an issue that needs to get sorted quickly.

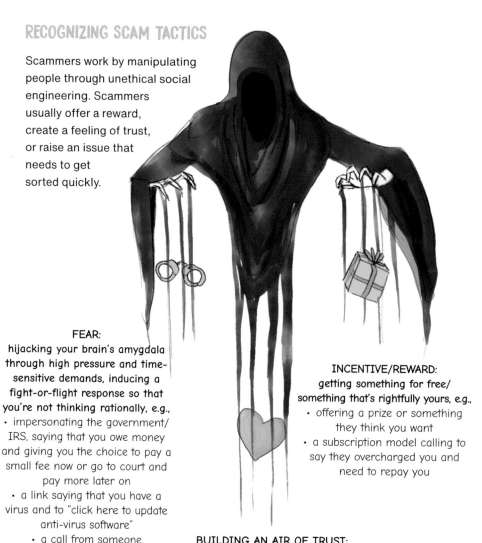

FEAR:
hijacking your brain's amygdala through high pressure and time-sensitive demands, inducing a fight-or-flight response so that you're not thinking rationally, e.g.,
- impersonating the government/ IRS, saying that you owe money and giving you the choice to pay a small fee now or go to court and pay more later on
- a link saying that you have a virus and to "click here to update anti-virus software"
- a call from someone impersonating a reputable tech-support company, saying that you have a virus
- a company saying your credit card has been compromised and you need to confirm your card details

INCENTIVE/REWARD:
getting something for free/ something that's rightfully yours, e.g.,
- offering a prize or something they think you want
- a subscription model calling to say they overcharged you and need to repay you

BUILDING AN AIR OF TRUST:
by sounding convincing and legitimate, e.g.,
- impersonating your phone provider and wanting to confirm your personal information to get as many details as possible to share with other scammers

HOW TO SPOT AND AVOID SCAMS

Warning
if you're being time-pressured into doing something

Warning
if you're being pressured not to hang up on a call

Warning
if someone asks for your password over the phone

LOOK OUT

Reminder
don't simply rely on the caller ID/email addresses/official-looking letters—scammers and hackers can impersonate those, too

Advice
confirm the person's identity by asking for information from them that only you and that provider should know

Advice
if something doesn't feel right, stop, ask to call back, search for the official phone number, call back from there, and then talk to someone you trust

THE IMPORTANCE OF PRIVACY

With new technology comes the opportunity for people to exploit you. They may be looking to gather information about you and your friends—for data collection, personal information, or passwords.

1. **Edit your social-media posts** that contain details about you: where you live and so on.
2. **Use a virtual private network (VPN)**, a service that protects your privacy online by hiding your IP address (virtual location) and encrypting your data, so that third parties—including internet providers—can't track your activity.
3. **Avoid oversharing personal and financial information** where it's not needed, especially on social media—question why someone needs your date of birth, for example. You can download Facebook data to see what it knows about you.
4. **Use messaging apps with end-to-end encryption**, such as Signal, so that messages can't be intercepted.

One final thing to say: hackers and scammers can be masters in security and social engineering, so don't feel silly if it happens to you.

WHAT SELF-DEFENSE ADVICE SHOULD I KNOW?

When you think of self-defense, do you think about spinning kicks and somersaults? While that may be great for some, it often requires high levels of fitness and being able-bodied. There is also an undertone of victim blaming: that if someone was attacked, assaulted, or raped, it was their fault, and if only they'd done a self-defense class they could have protected themselves. What were they wearing? Did they park next to a van? Were they walking home alone?

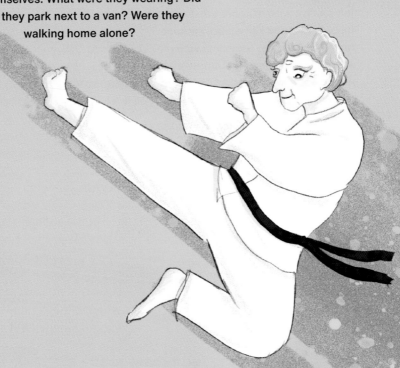

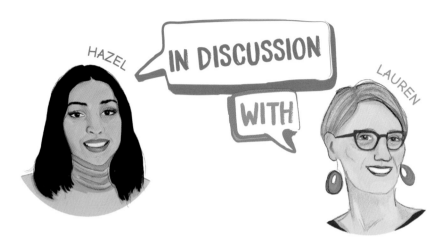

HAZEL

IN DISCUSSION WITH

LAUREN

The truth is that people get attacked in broad daylight, and in their own home, at work, or at school, and often the perpetrator is someone they know. There is a place for equipping yourself with skills so that you feel safer and more empowered, and that's where the self-defense organization Defend Yourself comes in. I interviewed its founder, Lauren R. Taylor, to get some advice and tips from a trauma-informed, non-victim-blaming angle.

Is there a way to recognize a threat?

Look at the other person's behavior. What are they doing that might be problematic? Whether that's something they're saying, or their body language, there are signs you can notice. Also, it helps to be in touch with our own feelings (how do I feel when I'm around this person?) and our own intuition. If you're a socialized female, you're oftentimes taught to put other people's feelings first, or not to hurt other people's feelings, or to generally people-please. So it's a practice of getting back in touch with your own feelings and intuition, slowing it down enough to check in with yourself and say, "How do I feel in this moment?" Respect it and respond, instead of just thinking, "Oh, it's probably nothing." Common physical signs are feeling a tightening in the chest, feeling uneasy in your gut, or feeling your palms getting sweaty.

If in a shocking situation you discover you have a freeze response, how can this be tackled?

The actual freeze is usually very short. You go into fight, flight, or freeze because your nervous system is overwhelmed. Take a class or practice on your own or with friends. If you feel you have more skills and more options, you're less likely to feel overwhelmed. Also, when you're in a freeze, you're probably not breathing. If you breathe, that can help break the freeze. When you're in a situation that you feel safe in—whether it's in your home, or you're with a friend you trust—imagine a stressful situation: maybe street harassment or something that puts some stress on you, but that isn't completely overwhelming. Feel that stress in your body, and breathe. Do that over and over, to where breathing becomes part of the programmed pattern.

Of course, the problem is not not just stranger-danger. It's everyday scenarios, too. Would there be anything you'd recommend in dealing with abusive family members or co-workers?

The vast majority of attacks on women and girls, and on LGBTQIA+ and non-binary people, are by people we know. Even if you're talking about sexual violence, the aggressors are most likely to be partners or exes. The next most common category is acquaintances, which includes friends, neighbors, co-workers. After that are other family members besides partners, and then the last category is people you don't know. It's helpful to pay attention to the way people in your life treat you. How am I feeling when they talk over me, or use a pet name that I told them that I don't like? Or when they tell me I'm making too big a deal about something? Or when they make fun of me, or criticize me a lot—all those relatively "little" things? These have their own power to violate and diminish us, and they're precursors to escalation. No abuse starts with hitting.

What do you think is the one thing that people don't think about, but really should, when it comes to self-defense?

Most people think they can't do it. And I want them to think they can, because it's true. You don't have to be fit. You don't have to be able-bodied. You don't have to commit yourself to years of study of the martial arts. Everybody can't do everything, but everybody can do something. ■

ARE THERE A COUPLE OF PHYSICAL DEFENSE MOVES THAT YOU COULD SHARE?

WHATEVER YOU'RE DOING, IF IT'S A PHYSICAL ATTACK, ALWAYS HAVE YOUR HANDS UP, IN A SOFT POSITION. THIS GIVES THE NON-VERBAL MESSAGE OF STOP, WHICH IS UNIVERSAL. AND IT'S ALSO THERE TO PROTECT YOU. YOU'RE READY TO ACT IF YOU NEED TO PROTECT YOUR HEAD.

ONE TIP IS TO MAKE A FIST BY FOLDING YOUR HANDS FINGERS DOWN, PUT YOUR THUMB ON THE OUTSIDE. THAT'S THE SAFEST WAY FOR YOU TO MAKE A FIST.

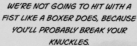

WE'RE NOT GOING TO HIT WITH A FIST LIKE A BOXER DOES, BECAUSE YOU'LL PROBABLY BREAK YOUR KNUCKLES.

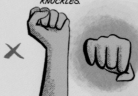

IT'S CALLED A HAMMER FIST. SO YOU WANT TO THINK OF YOURSELF LIKE YOU'RE HAMMERING OR LIKE YOU'RE A JUDGE WITH A GAVEL. THERE ARE LOTS OF DIFFERENT PLACES YOU CAN USE THIS –IT'S SO VERSATILE.

TAKE YOUR HAMMER FIST, AND ONE THING YOU CAN DO WITH IT IS TO HIT DOWN ON THE PERSON'S NOSE.

DOINK!

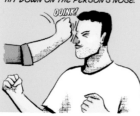

YOU CAN ALSO GO TO THE SIDES OF THE HEAD, TO THE TEMPLES.

STRAIGHT INTO THE THROAT.

TO MAKE SURE THAT YOU FEEL REALLY CONFIDENT WITH IT, WE EMPHASIZE USING YOUR WHOLE BODY POWER.

IF YOU'RE SITTING OR YOU USE A WHEELCHAIR, OR IF YOU END UP ON THE GROUND, YOU CAN ALSO HIT TO THEIR KNEE.

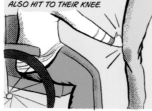

Let's say they're grabbing you, you can bring it down on the back of their hand.

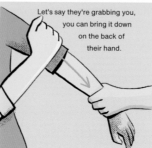

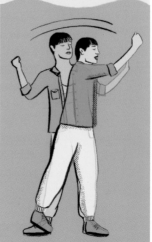

AND THE WAY I'M REALLY GOING TO GET EVEN MORE POWER IS THAT WHENEVER WE HIT, WE YELL.................

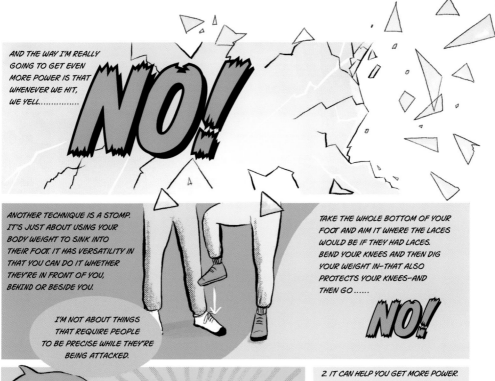

NO!

ANOTHER TECHNIQUE IS A STOMP. IT'S JUST ABOUT USING YOUR BODY WEIGHT TO SINK INTO THEIR FOOT. IT HAS VERSATILITY IN THAT YOU CAN DO IT WHETHER THEY'RE IN FRONT OF YOU, BEHIND OR BESIDE YOU.

I'M NOT ABOUT THINGS THAT REQUIRE PEOPLE TO BE PRECISE WHILE THEY'RE BEING ATTACKED.

TAKE THE WHOLE BOTTOM OF YOUR FOOT AND AIM IT WHERE THE LACES WOULD BE IF THEY HAD LACES. BEND YOUR KNEES AND THEN DIG YOUR WEIGHT IN—THAT ALSO PROTECTS YOUR KNEES—AND THEN GO ......

NO!

WHY THE YELLING?

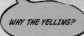

5 REASONS FOR YELLING

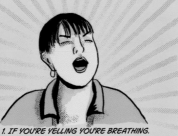

1. IF YOU'RE YELLING YOU'RE BREATHING.

2. IT CAN HELP YOU GET MORE POWER. YOU'VE SEEN THE WILLIAMS SISTERS WHEN THEY HIT, OR THE GUYS IN THE GYM.

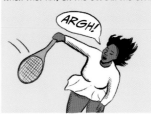

ARGH!

3. IT REINFORCES THAT YOUR MESSAGE IS "NO" OR "LEAVE ME ALONE."

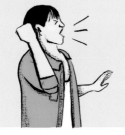

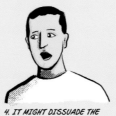

4. IT MIGHT DISSUADE THE ATTACKER BECAUSE SOMEONE MIGHT HEAR.

5. IT COULD BRING ATTENTION AND HELP.

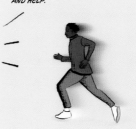

HOW DO I THINK CRITICALLY?

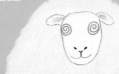

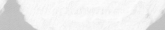

WHAT IS CRITICAL THINKING?

Critical thinking is self-guided thinking that seeks to be rational, to remove bias, and to understand how flawed human thought patterns can be, because the brain is highly susceptible to biases, ego, and emotion, which can cloud our judgment to see objectively.

A critical thinker:
- raises questions, rather than following blindly
- gathers information and assesses what concepts may be at work in the information provided
- can think open-mindedly and explore other points of view

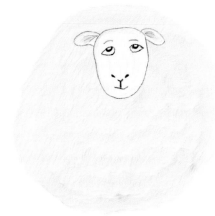

WHY IS CRITICAL THINKING DIFFICULT?

This is the first time that society has found itself with a wealth of information at its fingertips online. Previously we would have had to rely on what the authorities told us, without any way to do our own research and come to our own conclusions. Now a quick Google search can find an answer to any question.

Unfortunately, there is a danger, in that not everything you read online is true. Our biases lead us to research things that confirm what we *think* is true, rather than the truth. We are more likely to click on a video that is in line with our way of thinking than on one with the opposing view, and we are more likely to follow people on social media who align with our values than those who don't. This is "confirmation bias," and social-media platforms and search engines don't necessarily help. Their aim is to show us content that will keep us using them for longer, so algorithms suggest similar items that align with the views we've already shown a preference for. Many newspapers lean left or right, so you're more likely to get a non-neutral viewpoint on the news by reading them, rather than an unbiased look at the facts.

HOW TO IMPROVE CRITICAL THINKING

1

RECOGNIZE CONFIRMATION BIAS:
we are more likely to accept something as evidence if it agrees with our point of view. If we're willing to change our minds, we are likely to be more open to all information.

2

CHECK YOUR SOURCE:
is it reliable, and how is the data being presented? Data can be biased, too. Could there be any ulterior motives?

3

RECOGNIZE AND AVOID LOGICAL FALLACIES IN ARGUMENTS (SEE OPPOSITE PAGE):
notice when others are using them to make points, and avoid using them yourself when arguing and debating with others.

4

UNDERSTAND NUANCE AND COMPLEXITY:
social media doesn't encourage long-form or in-depth discussions, especially with short tweets, short TikToks, or in an Instagram square. While there's a place for that, it's important to recognize that topics get condensed and simplified to black and white. Often topics aren't that simple.

5

LET GO OF THE NEED TO BE RIGHT:
or be receptive to the idea that you might be wrong.

6

TRY TO ACTIVELY FIND OPPOSING VIEWPOINTS:
this can strengthen your point of view or even change or soften it.

A LOOK AT LOGICAL FALLACIES

Logical fallacies are flawed, deceptive reasonings that are used in arguments to make something seem more persuasive than it is. There are plenty of them, but here are a few.

 STRAW MAN a misrepresentation of someone's view, which distorts or exaggerates someone's argument so that it's easier to attack

 APPEAL TO IGNORANCE argues that a proposition/conclusion must be true because there is no evidence against it; this shifts the need for proof away

 AD HOMINEM relying on personal attacks to undermine someone's argument—think mudslinging in politics to sway voters, rather than concrete points

 APPEAL TO AUTHORITY misusing an authority's opinion in place of an actual argument

 SLIPPERY SLOPE implies a certain course of action will lead to a catastrophic chain of events, based on tenuous links, so that attention is shifted to those hypotheticals

 HASTY GENERALIZATION an argument that uses a few examples rather than substantial proof; if it's true in a couple of cases, then it must be true in all cases

 BANDWAGON implies that something must be true because others believe it, even though people can be mistaken

 APPEAL TO HYPOCRISY focusing on a person's hypocrisy to distract from the issue, avoiding having to engage with criticism by turning it back on the accuser

 RED HERRING makes an irrelevant argument to distract attention towards a different topic and false conclusion

Conclusion: My Life Lessons

I hope you've found these pages and words helpful—and that even just one person feels more seen as they close this book.

Reflecting on the lessons I learned in school, and all the stats and facts I've discovered while writing this, I realize that we are more often taught how to memorize, rather than how to question and interrogate what we're being told or to think critically. We can't believe everything we're told or everything we see, or even everything we remember—our memories are skewed and can be tricked (think about when you and your parents have a very different recollection of how an event happened). When we're younger we have such curiosity and questioning, but when we settle into our views and ourselves, we can lose that curiosity, instead feeling comfortable in the fact that we are "right."

Using critical thinking, we can digest information we are fed, and dissect it, understanding that the world around us is much more nuanced than we're led to believe. We can get to the bottom of why different societal myths have been enforced on us and free ourselves from the shame that these sometimes harmful beliefs have embedded within us.

It's easy to believe everyone should think the same as we do, and want the same things out of life we do, but we're all different, and this is where empathy—another crucial lesson—comes into play.

When we put ourselves into someone else's shoes we can be more open-minded and understand different perspectives. When people are reduced to statistics or stereotypes it's easy to dehumanize them, but listening to others and talking face to face, with eye contact (rather than on a screen), can allow us to be less judgmental, less immediately prickly towards strangers, and to remember that they're human, too. Empathy is also key in terms of navigating relationships with partners, family, and colleagues, where you have to consider the feelings of others and be able to discuss and compromise in places where you may not see eye to eye.

In addition to the questions I've explored in this book, I want to leave you with some final thoughts—some life lessons that I've learned throughout my short time on this Earth, which you can take or leave:

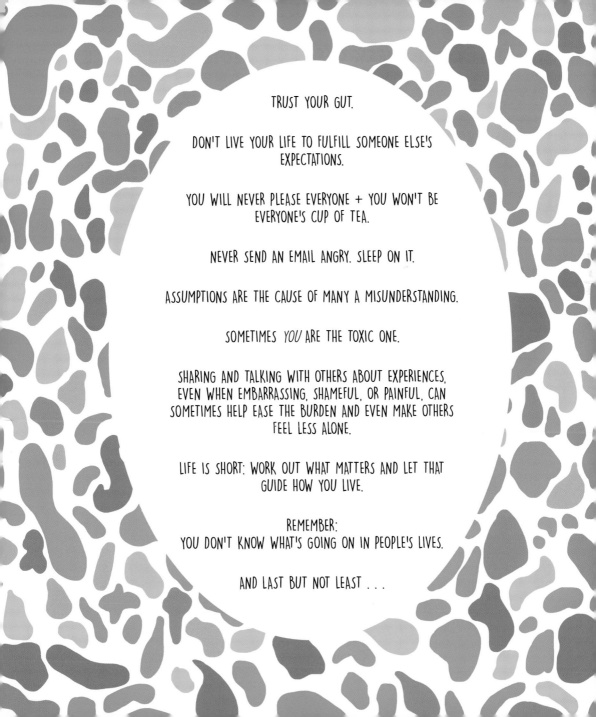

TRUST YOUR GUT.

DON'T LIVE YOUR LIFE TO FULFILL SOMEONE ELSE'S
EXPECTATIONS.

YOU WILL NEVER PLEASE EVERYONE + YOU WON'T BE
EVERYONE'S CUP OF TEA.

NEVER SEND AN EMAIL ANGRY. SLEEP ON IT.

ASSUMPTIONS ARE THE CAUSE OF MANY A MISUNDERSTANDING.

SOMETIMES *YOU* ARE THE TOXIC ONE.

SHARING AND TALKING WITH OTHERS ABOUT EXPERIENCES,
EVEN WHEN EMBARRASSING, SHAMEFUL, OR PAINFUL, CAN
SOMETIMES HELP EASE THE BURDEN AND EVEN MAKE OTHERS
FEEL LESS ALONE.

LIFE IS SHORT: WORK OUT WHAT MATTERS AND LET THAT
GUIDE HOW YOU LIVE.

REMEMBER:
YOU DON'T KNOW WHAT'S GOING ON IN PEOPLE'S LIVES.

AND LAST BUT NOT LEAST . . .

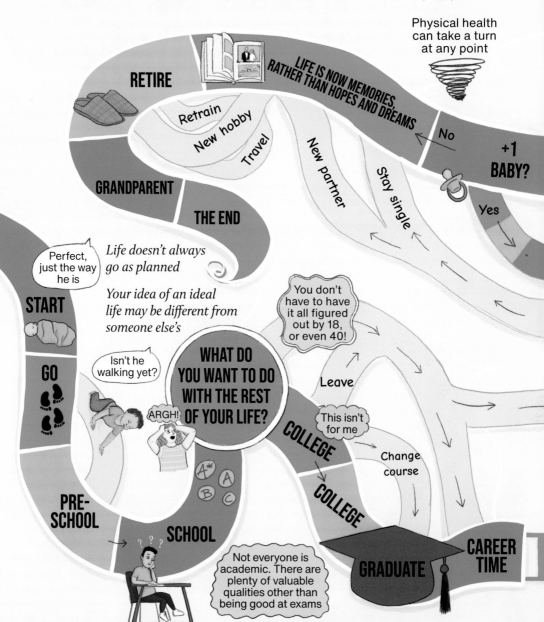

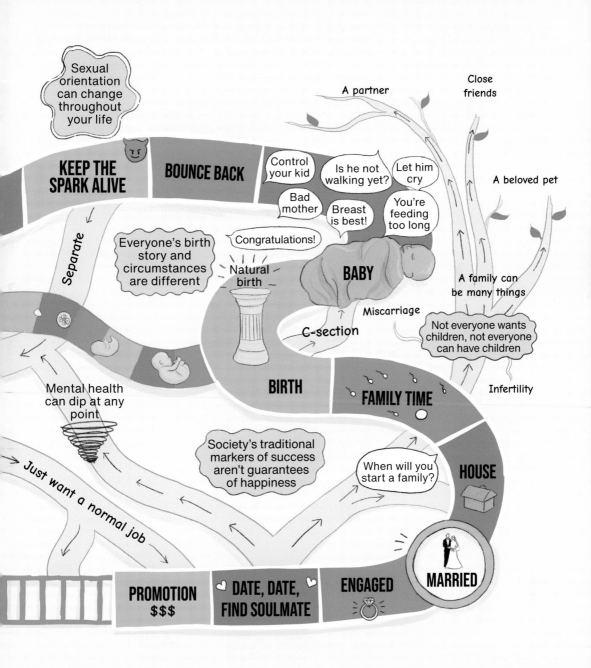

Sources

Introduction: Banana + Condom + Shame = Sex Ed

Google search trends are taken from Google's own 'Year in Search' statistics. The most-searched mental health terms come from the marketing firm Mondovo's research and from the World Economic Forum.

Relationships + Sex

Statistics on the prevalence of domestic violence are from the National Institutes of Health (NIH) and the National Domestic Violence Hotline.

The discovery of the first vertebrate fish mother 380 million years ago was recorded by Live Science.

The study "Virginity Testing: A Systematic Review" was conducted by Rose McKeon Olson and Claudia García-Moreno and published in Reproductive Health.

The "hymen myth" was based on Natural Cycles' article "5 Hymen Facts You Should Know."

The quotes from Lynn Enright are from an interview on womanandhome.com.

Vaginal discharge cycle information is based on articles by Clue, Medical News Today, and the NHS. Information about vaginal odor

is from a Healthline article which quotes guidance from Felice Gersh. Penis myths are busted in J. Shah and N. Christopher's study "Can Shoe Size Predict Penile Length?"; in Medical News Today, "10 Things You Didn't Know About the Penis"; and in the NHS article "Is It Normal to Have a Curved Penis?"

The definition of "intersex" is based on the Intersex Society of North America's own definition.

The G spot study and the orgasm gap studies mentioned are titled "Does the G-spot Exist? A Review of the Current Literature" (Vincenzo Puppo and Ilan Gruenwald) and "Differences in Orgasm Frequency Among Gay, Lesbian, Bisexual, and Heterosexual Men and Women in a U.S. National sample" (David A. Frederick, H. Kate St John, Justin R. Garcia, Elisabeth A. Lloyd).

Information about female discomfort from prolonged arousal without orgasm can be found at health.com.

The lube infographic includes advice from Healthline, The Femedic, Metro, Clue, and Hart's Desires.

Contraception stats and information comes from the NHS website, Contraception Choices, and Planned Parenthood. The information about PrEP comes from Prepster.

Sexuality and romance terminology is based on the University of Connecticut Rainbow Center's LGBTQIA+ Dictionary, and Healthline's article "What Does It Mean to Be Sexually Fluid?"

The definition of consent is from the website RAINN. Statistics on rape convictions are from Ballotpedia, RAINN, and the FBI's website.

Health + Wellbeing

The chart on recognizing negative thought patterns is based on information by Sage Neuroscience Center.

Socrates' musings on self-care (among other things!) were recorded by Plato and are widely reproduced.

The biology of stress is inspired by research laid out in Robert M. Sapolsky's book Why Zebras Don't Get Ulcers and the illustration of stress in the body takes inspiration from Psychology Today's article "Where Do You Store Stress in Your Body? Top 10 Secret Areas."

The "grief in different cultures" illustration is inspired by an article in The Conversation.

The information on impact bias is based on Dan Gilbert's TED Talk, "The Surprising Science of Happiness."

The jam experiment mentioned is titled "When Choice Is

Demotivating: Can One Desire Too Much of a Good Thing?" (Sheena S. Iyengar and Mark R. Lepper).

Information on the menstrual cycle itself, and what is normal, is provided by the MSD Manual and NHS Inform. Information on menstrual cycle phases and color comes from Clue.

Statistics for the infographic on medical bias come from studies on gender discrepancies in abdominal pain tratment by Chen et al., and Siddiqui et. al.; a meta-analysis on pain treatment disparities in tie US by Salimah et. al.; a study on racial disparities in pain mangement by Mossey; a UK study on representation in medical research by Smart and Harrison; studies in gender differences in heart disease by Kyker and Limacher, Løvlien, Schei, and Gjengedal; and Majidi et al.; an ACVC article on heart attaches by Wu et. al; and a 1997 study on problems in accurate medical diagnosis of depression in female patients by Floyd.

Guidance around the signs and symptoms of breast cancer and how to check your breasts is based on advice from CoppaFeel, and guidance around the signs and symptoms of testicular cancer and how to check your balls is based on advice from Prostate Cancer UK.

The Self + Society

Neurodivergent terms are based on descriptions provided by Autism Speaks, the National Institute of Neurological Disorders and Stroke, the NHS, MedicineNet, the British Dyslexia Association, DSF Literacy and Clinical Services, and WebMD.

Digital security tips are based on information by the Federal Trade Commission: Consumer Advice and from the cybersecurity firm Cipher. The logical fallacies are based on the website yourlogicalfallacyis.com.

Further Reading

Advice and support are available if you are dealing with an abusive relationship:

The National Domestic Violence Hotline: www.thehotline.org

Love is Respect: loveisrespect.org

If you have been sexually assaulted you can contact RAINN at www. rainn.org/resources

Some references for seeing and appreciating the diversity of genitalia:

The Great Wall of Vagina by Jamie McCartney

100 Vaginas, a Channel 4 documentary about 100 vulvas, and their stories by photographer Laura Dodsworth

Manhood: The Bare Reality by Laura Dodsworth

Vagina: A Re-Education by Lynn Enright

For more comprehensive advice on how to prepare for a cervical screening, please visit The Eve Appeal and Jo's Cervical Cancer Trust.

For further advice and support for ADHD I would suggest the YouTube channel How to ADHD.

Glossary

Agricultural revolution: the transition from a hunter-gatherer society to one of settled agriculture; the first agricultural revolution occurred c.10,000 BCE

Amygdala: the almond-shaped region of the brain associated with emotional processes

Body neutrality: being focused on accepting and appreciating what your body can do

Body positivity: feeling good towards and loving your own body (and others' bodies)

Boundaries: the parameters of what you're okay with and what you're not

Cervix: the lower part of the uterus

Cognitive behavioral therapy (CBT): a talking therapy that focuses on changing the way you think and behave

Contentment: an emotional state of satisfaction; a milder but perhaps longer-lasting state than happiness

Encryption: the conversion of information or data that's readable into something that's encoded

End-to-end encryption: a secure communication that prevents others from accessing data in the transmission process from one system to another

Enthusiastic consent: a clear, positive, excited "yes" in response to an offer

Fawn response: appeasing someone else in order to diffuse and avoid conflict

Grief: intense sadness due to loss, especially death

Happiness: a positive, pleasant emotional state of joy

Human papillomavirus (HPV): a common group of viruses that affect the skin, spread through skin-to-skin genital contact, sex, or sharing toys; for most people, HPV doesn't cause symptoms, but for some it can cause genital warts or cell changes, which can sometimes turn cancerous

Identity crisis: a period of confusion when someone's idea of who they are gets overturned or fractured, often due to the catalyst of role change or upheaval

Living loss: grief without a death

Malware: computer software that has been designed to damage or interfere with a system

Materialism: the desire to own lots of possessions or money

Microaggression: everyday verbal or behavioral slights that show negative or derogatory attitudes towards marginalized groups; often unintentionally offensive

Mindfulness: a state of awareness, observation, and acceptance, especially concerned with the present moment

Misogyny: a strong prejudice or hatred towards women

Nervous system: this includes the brain, the spinal cord, and a network of nerve tissue that transmits signals from the brain to the rest of the body

Nuance: a subtle distinction that may be difficult to see, but important to note

Rape: unlawful sexual activity, intercourse, or sexual penetration without the consent of the other person, or with an individual who is incapable of giving consent due to intoxication, unconsciousness, deception, being a minor, or mental illness

Red flag: a warning sign that shows manipulation or unhealthy behavior

Revenge porn: the sharing of private sexual material of someone without their consent and with the purpose of causing embarrassment

Sex: may be vaginal, anal, or oral; stimulation of the genitals and masturbation can also be considered under the umbrella of sex

Social engineering: psychologically manipulating users into giving away personal information that may be used for fraudulent purposes

Spontaneous desire: a spark that

seems to arise out of the blue
Two-factor authentication:
a computer security system
that requires users to provide
two different ways to verify
themselves as the correct user
Upskirting: taking a photo under
someone's clothing without
their consent
Vagina: the internal canal that
connects the cervix of the
uterus to external genitalia
Virus: a type of malware that
can attach itself, copy itself,
and infect a computer
Vulva: the outer part of the
female genitals
Wellbeing: a state of comfort,
happiness, and health

Acknowledgments

When you let go of the egotistical need to do everything yourself, and collaborate with people, magic happens. Thank you to the talented team that has worked on shaping this book into something much better than I could have created on my own. I have to mention Sophie, Mylène, Emily, Bryony, Graeme, and Mandy for their dedication and smart ideas.

A special thank you to Marianne for believing in me and this idea from the very start, and for her kindness, compassion, and creativity throughout this process.

To my closest friends and family, thank you for eternally supporting me, for never doubting my illustration career—even when I did—and for bearing with me this year while I've been MIA.

To Ryszard, who is the most wonderfully supportive partner I could have asked for, who was always there when I needed someone to soundboard ideas, helped me through when I was struggling, and very excitedly advised on the digital security chapter. I love you.

And finally, for younger me, younger siblings of mine, and for friends—this book was written for you!

HAZEL MEAD
IS AN ILLUSTRATOR WHO COMES FROM
A FAMILY OF ARTISTS. KNOWN FOR HER VIRAL
ILLUSTRATIONS DEMYSTIFYING PERIODS, POINTING
OUT SEXISM, AND INVITING US TO LOOK AT EACH
OTHER WITH EMPATHY, HAZEL'S WORK SHOWCASES
DIVERSITY AND INVITES US ALL TO SEE OTHERS WITH
AN OPEN MIND AND TO THINK CRITICALLY ABOUT
STEREOTYPES IN THE MEDIA. SHE LIKES TO USE
HER ART TO START CONVERSATIONS AND QUESTION
TABOOS AND SOCIAL NORMS TO HELP EVERYONE
FEEL LIKE THEY CAN BE THEMSELVES.

SHE CAN BE FOUND ON
INSTAGRAM AS
@HAZEL.MEAD

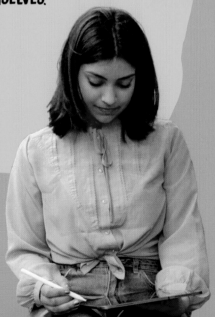

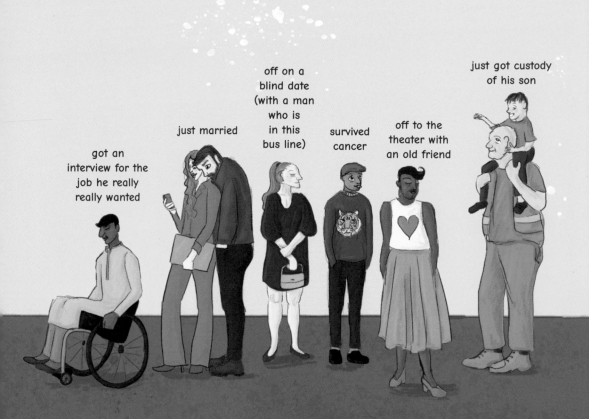